"Rapid technological change is fast-tracking the of digital innovations in applied psychological ɪ have dramatically increased the digitisation of tɪ and services ranging from psychodiagnostics to .... These innovations aim to scale the availability of psychological services and increase accessibility for traditionally marginalised communities. Arguably the COVID-19 pandemic furthermore made these digital psychological services more than a novelty and has established them as the norm. Psychological practitioners have adopted new technological approaches to their assessment and development practices to compensate for the barriers COVID-19 restrictions have placed on their traditional approaches to practice. However, are we aware of the challenges this new way of work poses to our practices and our clients? Do we know the risks that this new way of work poses for our clients' safety, security, and psychological wellbeing? And are our practices prepared for managing the risks associated with digital mental health services?

In her new book, Alexandra explores the contemporary challenges, risks, and ethical dilemmas that digital mental health services pose to data security and client welfare. Specifically, she provides a practitioner-friendly guide for managing digital client data, mitigating risks and securing your practice against cybercrime. Her book further attempts to enhance practitioners' digital competence to ensure that you have a future-fit, resilient and digitally secured practice. This book is a 'must' for any therapist, psychologist, or coach venturing into the world of digital mental health."

Professor Dr Llewellyn van Zyl, *Extraordinary Professor in Positive Psychology, NWU*

"This book is a must-have for any coach, therapist or organisations handling sensitive data whose eyes glaze over when the word 'cybersecurity' is mentioned! It's jam-packed with information and tips to ensure you're safely and securely protecting your business and your clients' confidentiality and information. It also helps you create a trusted and safe environment, which is the foundation of a strong client relationship."

Dr Suzy Green, *DPsych (Clin) MAPS, The Positivity Institute – Founder & CEO*

"Nobody expects to be the victim of cybercrime or defrauded. Yet thousands become victims of cybercriminals each day. Imagine the feeling if criminals steal and leak your clients' biggest secrets? The good news is that you can help prevent it from happening by reading this book. Alexandra, both a coach and cyber fraud expert herself, provides actionable and proven tips on how to ensure that you will not become the next victim of the criminals. Read this book – and learn from one of the best!"

Mindaugas Kutkaitis, *Fraud Prevention Expert, Financial Services*

important message, that good digital hygiene is becoming less about raw technology and more about a holistic, defensive mindset."

Sean Henley, *Technology Strategy &*
Resilience Manager, Financial Services

"Cybersecurity . . . oftentimes people will get intimidated by this term. That is something for the 'IT Expert' to sort out, not me. No one will actually try to attack my information or account. That is for the 'big companies'. That is a misconception this book will help clear up. It really can happen to us all. With the tools and information given to you in this book, you will realise there is in fact a lot you can do yourself. The book will also show, you do not need to be an 'IT Expert' to secure yourself and your business. Take the opportunity to read this book. It will be an eye opener."

H. Erik Inberg, *Senior Technical Manager,*
Support & Projects

"This reassuring, practical and informative guide to coach and therapist cybersecurity, focused on how to protect client data, is long overdue. Alexandra has a knack of presenting, what could otherwise be a complicated diet of ideas, in a wholly digestible format. In straightforward, encouraging language, she raises practitioner awareness of potential issues, improving competence and confidence in preventing fraud, promoting security online, carefully considering ethical practice and always looking for the best outcomes for both practitioner and client. Every coach and therapist needs to read this book."

Ruth Hughes, *Course Director, Cambridge*
Coaching Certificate Programme

"Understanding the psychology behind cybersecurity is to understand one of the biggest threats to the economical world as we know it today. As a cybersecurity professional, I have at first hand seen not only how well organised and imposing cyberattacks can be on enterprises but also how intimidating and debilitating it can be for people. One thing is the loss of money, the other and most important thing is the impact it has on a human psyche, and how it can ruin lives, relationships and trust in the human race. Putting in place good cybersecurity is then the stepping stone for securing your practices and keeping clients safe."

Kim Ottobrøker, *Compliance Specialist, Danish Utility Sector*

"Fraud and cybercrime are increasing problems, impacting all areas of society, and putting organisations as well as individuals at risk. Today, no one is safe, and anyone can become a target of criminals operating on a global scale. In this highly relevant book on cybersecurity, Alexandra J.S. Fouracres shares her extensive knowledge about the subject with the reader and gives a thorough introduction to the concepts and how criminals operate. This book is highly recommended, as it provides the reader with the necessary tools and knowledge needed to avoid becoming a victim of fraud and cybercrime."

Kristian E. Stephansen, *Card Fraud Prevention Expert*

Cybersecurity for Coaches and Therapists

This groundbreaking book filters down the wealth of information on cybersecurity to the most relevant and highly applicable aspects for coaches, therapists, researchers and all other practitioners handling confidential client conversations and data.

Whether working with clients online or face to face, practitioners today increasingly rely on the cyberspace as part of their practice. Through a solutions-focused lens, the book provides easy-to-apply practical advice and guidelines using non-technical language, enabling practitioners to mitigate the rising threat of cybercrime, which can no longer be ignored. By the last page the reader will have knowledge and awareness towards: securing devices, spotting financial fraud, mitigating the risks of online communications, operating more securely from a home office and handling a cyber event if one occurs.

Clear, concise, and easy to follow, this guide is a pivotal resource for coaches, therapists, researchers and all other practitioners protecting their clients and businesses.

Alexandra J.S. Fouracres is a cybersecurity manager and cyber fraud expert in addition to working as a coaching psychologist, academic and published researcher. She holds qualifications in coaching psychology and positive psychology and is a member of the British Psychological Society.

Cybersecurity for Coaches and Therapists

A Practical Guide for Protecting Client Data

Alexandra J.S. Fouracres

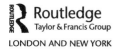
Routledge
Taylor & Francis Group

LONDON AND NEW YORK

Cover image: Getty Images

First published 2022
by Routledge
4 Park Square, Milton Park, Abingdon, Oxon OX14 4RN

and by Routledge
605 Third Avenue, New York, NY 10158

Routledge is an imprint of the Taylor & Francis Group, an informa business

British Library Cataloguing-in-Publication Data
A catalogue record for this book is available from the British Library

Library of Congress Cataloging-in-Publication Data
Names: Fouracres, Alexandra J. S., author.
Title: Cybersecurity for coaches and therapists : a practical guide for protecting client data / Alexandra J.S. Fouracres.
Description: Abingdon, Oxon ; New York, NY : Routledge, 2022. | Includes bibliographical references and index. | Summary: "This ground-breaking book distills the wealth of information on cybersecurity to the most relevant and highly applicable aspects for coaches, therapists, researchers and all practitioners handling client-confidential conversations and data"— Provided by publisher.
Identifiers: LCCN 2021051844 | ISBN 9781032027173 (hardback) | ISBN 9781032027166 (paperback) | ISBN 9781003184805 (ebook)
Subjects: LCSH: Psychiatric records—Access control. | Psychiatric records—Data processing. | Computer security. | Data protection.
Classification: LCC RC455.2.M38 F88 2022 | DDC 616.8900285—dc23/eng/20220111
LC record available at https://lccn.loc.gov/2021051844

ISBN: 978-1-032-02717-3 (hbk)
ISBN: 978-1-032-02716-6 (pbk)
ISBN: 978-1-003-18480-5 (ebk)

DOI: 10.4324/9781003184805

Typeset in Times New Roman
by Apex CoVantage, LLC

In memory of Eric John Fouracres

Contents

Foreword

"Cybersecurity" – in the past this phrase could have been construed as an armed force pulled together by the federation to protect from the attacks of marauding cyborgs. However, cybersecurity is most definitely not a work of fiction nor is it something belonging to the future. It is very much a need and issue of the present day.

In many cases, though, it is still seen as the preserve of large global organisations with IT departments and technology officers holding tons of secret sauce in their IT systems that they do not want anyone else getting their greedy cyber hands on. At the same time, the reality, in this day and age, is that personal data is in as much demand, if not more, as any industrial secret sauce. Furthermore, because of the large-scale resources available to any sizeable organisation and their ability to monitor and protect their systems in an automated fashion, attention and focus have shifted to the more vulnerable. The sole practitioner who has confidential client data in a spreadsheet or some off-the-shelf client management system – where protocols around patching, updating and virus protection software are likely to be more haphazard and infrequent – may be considered a softer and easier target. There is also an element of using the smaller provider as a backdoor into the global organisations and their larger databases.

We owe it to ourselves, our clients and others who entrust us with their data to ensure that it is stored safely and in a protected manner. For that, we must know and understand how we protect our devices and the data that is stored on them. At times, for the non-technical, the information can be too techy, overwhelming and difficult to get to grips with and follow. That is why this book is an absolute treasure, as Alexandra identifies the threats that we need to be aware of and provides practical and pragmatic ways in which our devices and files can be protected against those threats. Drawing on her extensive experience in cyber fraud, alongside her training as a coaching psychologist, Alexandra walks the reader through the steps, building and reinforcing as she goes. For those who doubt the need, she has also included enough examples of how storing and safe-guarding personal data, and in particular sensitive personal data, of others can go wrong and what happens when it does, to persuade them otherwise.

Providing practical suggestions and advice, along with some concluding check-lists, this book will both persuade you of the absolute need to improve the level of security that you already apply and encourage you to reassess on a regular basis. The cybercriminals are a creative bunch who don't sit still for long; therefore, those of us who wish to protect our data from them cannot afford to do so either.

By Samantha Fletcher-Watts, PC. dp, FCA Ireland

Preface

The media stories and the complex volumes of materials that have been written up about cybercrime and fraud have meant people have become more aware. However, the complexity of the information often means people also continue to look forward, blinkers on, and hope cybercrime won't happen to them. Those that work with the victims see that it does.

The truth is that technology keeps evolving, and it is overdue that we include cybersecurity as part of our ethics as practitioners. Being more aware of the risks out there, and putting into place some simple integrity practices around our data security, needs to be embedded into our day-to-day as practitioners in a technological age.

This book does this gradually, through building up information and knowledge as well as skills and comprehension. It might not be a surprise that as an author working with coaching psychology and positive psychology – as well as working in the subject field – that I have deliberately constructed the chapters to be solutions focused and enable new cognitive–behavioural pathways. This is done through building strengths, resilience and those all-important factors of competence and agency. By the last page, a new mindset towards cybersecurity is installed. The reader will no longer want to look away, but instead has already applied much of what has been learnt through small actions set for them, leaving them now better equipped and ready to absorb new information by themselves, going forward.

*

Perhaps to have contrast with all the different teams and groups I am in, this was a journey I simply decided to take quietly on my own. Thanks are still due to everyone in the writing group I have been part of some twenty years now, for ongoing wisdom that I have absorbed and support in the last months, even if I have not directly mentioned this project. Gratitude is also due to Samantha Fletcher-Watts, for being my sounding board, despite our different time-zones, and for being nothing but supportive and encouraging from start to end.

Thank you to everyone at Routledge – for understanding the vision of this book from the first moment.

Most of all, thank you to each reader coming on this journey that I hope will give you a new, more positive view of cybersecurity that you will take with you, going forward.

Acknowledgements

Crown copyright sources referenced in this book are licenced under the terms of the Open Government Licence v 3.0 (https://www.nationalarchives.gov.uk/doc /open-government-licence/version/3/).

Disclaimer

The information provided in this book is designed to provide information and motivation on the subjects discussed. Cybersecurity is a changing environment that this book cannot anticipate, nor can the approaches described herein protect each reader from every cyberthreat they may encounter. Neither the publisher nor the author shall be liable for any loss or damage caused to any person acting, as a result of the material in this publication.

This book is not meant to be used, nor should it be used, as a substitute for professional advice. Don't use the information contained in this book in place of relevant and necessary professional advice to assist you as needed with applying the topics covered, setting up a cybersecurity framework or managing a cybersecurity incident.

While best efforts have been used in preparing this book, the author and publisher make no representations or warranties of any kind, and assume no liabilities of any kind with respect to the accuracy or completeness of the contents and specifically disclaim any implied warranties of merchantability or fitness of use for a particular purpose.

The author and publisher are providing general advice and are not responsible for any specific unknown situation of the reader and are not liable for any damages or negative consequences from any action, application or decision, by any person reading or following the information in this book.

References are provided for informational purposes only and do not constitute endorsement of any websites, links, articles or other sources. All links are for information purposes only and are not warranted for content, accuracy or any other implied or explicit purpose. Readers should be aware that the websites, articles, links listed in this book may change or become unavailable.

Creating a secure practice

Cybersecurity isn't difficult. The problem is where to start, with so much overwhelming and alarming information out there.

This book provides you with a new view, simplifying a wealth of information on cybersecurity and fraud down to what may be most urgently relevant to coaches, therapists, counsellors, psychologists, researchers and anyone else handling confidential client conversations and data.

Cybercrime and technology will continue to evolve, and criminals can strike at any time. However, this book guides you through what we do have control over:

Understanding the risks
Implementing good cybersecurity practices
Building a foundational understanding and competencies to take forward
Knowing how to react if something happens

By the last page, you will have put in place some simple, instant action points. You will be able to continue the path alone, with an understanding of the threats and vulnerabilities most applicable to your line of work, and how to mitigate and react to them. Your new cybersecurity ethical best practices will be part of your day-to-day, and you will have created an enhanced trusted environment for your client interactions and data.

Watch out though – by the end of this reading journey, some of you will learn to love researching combating cybercrime and fraud prevention. You might find yourself immersed in this new world!

Introduction

This book will enhance your ability to create a safe and trusted environment for your client and their data. The advice within is tailored specifically for coaches, therapists, psychologists, researchers, counsellors and all other practitioners handling confidential client data. The information is constructed as a practical learning experience. Through it, practitioners can incorporate simple foundations into their day-to-day, including secure storage of data, making informed choices about security tools and learning to spot the red flags of cybercrime. Overall enabling improved cyber resilience and formation of powerful habits around cybersecurity that can be built on, along with an ability to react if something happens.

Basic cybersecurity is not as difficult as we think it is. It just requires some reading, absorption and implementation. Much of the media around cybercrime can create a maelstrom of fear. Break it down, and it looks a little different: technology and security are topics that quite simply need an eye-catching headline to get people who don't work in those areas to read them! Without imposing headlines luring us in, many would likely still be uninformed about cybercrime, cyber fraud and the various ways criminals infiltrate businesses or private accounts to steal information and money.

Technology and its use will keep evolving; along with it, so will cyber risks. According to the US Secret Service (2020), the line between cybersecurity and financial crime has become increasingly entangled. The Office of National Statistics (ONS, 2021) in the United Kingdom published results from a telephone-operated crime survey conducted across England and Wales, revealing among other crimes an estimated 4.4 million fraud incidents and 1.7 million computer misuse incidents (such as hacking, viruses and malware) across the 12 months up to the end of September 2020. The threat is unfortunately very real. In March 2021, GOV.UK released results of a UK survey in which 39% of businesses had reported experiencing a cybersecurity breach or attack in the previous 12 months (Department for Digital, Culture, Media and Sport [DCMS], 2021). This, in a year, in which many businesses had a period of closure; it would be perhaps more pertinent to look at the figure from the year before, which was 46% (DCMS, 2020).

DOI: 10.4324/9781003184805-1

The data so far shows that everyone is a target for cybercriminals and fraud-sters, who continually evolve their capabilities. The occupation someone has is often less relevant than how open the door is left for a criminal to get in. That said, as we will cover later, the practitioners reading this book make for very interesting targets. Any business can be targeted for financial gain, but a practitioner with confidential data will also be targeted to obtain particularly lucrative sensitive data and thus more financial gain through blackmail or extortion.

The lines that criminals will cross to gain from cybercrime do not involve any concern for ethics, confidentiality and data security – these being the most fundamental requirements of a practitioner reading this book, who typically informs their clients that all their interactions are confidential. The message through all the chapters should become clear: cyberthreats are so prevalent that it is impossible to ensure confidentiality and data privacy without consciously implementing cybersecurity in practice.

For a practitioner working with confidential data, cybersecurity can help reduce the risk of the following issues for their practice:

- Damage to reputation due to breach of confidential data pertaining to clients, or from having to disclose a breach that has come from poor security or controls
- Loss of business/earnings due to either loss of reputation or disruption and downtime caused by a cyber event or fraud
- Financial loss due to a cyberattack or fraud
- Fines/penalties for not implementing any necessary data security measures in relation to local/national laws
- Consequences of breaching ethical conduct guidelines/codes of conduct of relevant accreditation and membership bodies or licencing boards related to topics such as ensuring confidentiality and correct data handling

Being more aware of the risks out there, and putting into place some simple integrity practices around our data security, then needs to be embedded into our ethical practice as practitioners in a technological age. Yet, the self-employed and small- and medium-sized businesses do not always have available to them the information they need to prevent, cope with or respond to a cyberthreat (Gafni & Pavel, 2019). This book will offer knowledge and practical solutions to address that issue.

While there is no silver bullet or one-step-fits-all to prevent cyberattacks, data breaches or fraud attempts, by the last page of this book, improved cyber practices and behaviours will be in place (which include due care to prevent an event and detect and react if one does occur). This making each practitioner reading this and applying the information less of a target for criminals and enabling them to say they are a more cybersecure practitioner who has added to their ethics toolkit actual security around their client data.

Your toolkit

The pages of this book build, among other things, the following toolkit:

Prevention and mitigation

- Active implementation (as you read) of best practices around cybersecurity to build your defences
- Case studies and knowledge on how to spot specific cyberthreats
- Information towards keeping computers and other electronic devices as secure as possible
- Advice on how to benchmark if you are using the most up-to-date and secure products available
- Tips on how to enhance the protection of stored client data
- Benefits of sharing with your client what you do in order to create a safe environment for their data and your interactions together
- Actions to lower the risk of fraud losses on your bank accounts

Awareness

- Understanding the specific cyberthreats and fraud types that pose a higher risk for the practitioners reading this book
- Recognising why good ethical practices around cybersecurity are required to fulfil ethics requirements around confidentiality and compliance with data privacy legislation
- Alertness as to the cyber risks of any software/tools
- Enhanced attentiveness to red flags, abnormalities and scams
- New appreciation of the importance of data security for both practitioner and client

Response ready

- Ability to respond quickly and competently to a security breach or cyberattack
- First possible steps – if you become a victim of cyber-enabled fraud
- Tips for recovery and moving forward

References

Department for Digital, Culture, Media and Sport (DCMS). (2020). *Cyber security breaches survey 2020*. Gov.UK. Crown Copyright. https://www.gov.uk/government/statistics/cyber-security-breaches-survey-2020
Department for Digital, Culture, Media and Sport (DCMS). (2021). *Cyber security skills in the UK labour market 2021*. Gov.UK. Crown Copyright. https://www.gov.uk/government/publications/cyber-security-skills-in-the-uk-labour-market-2021

Gafni, G., & Pavel, T. (2019). The invisible hole of information on SMB's cybersecurity. *Online Journal of Applied Knowledge Management (OJAKM)*, 7(1), 14–26. https://doi.org/10.36965/OJAKM.2019.7(1)

Office for National Statistics. (2021). *Crime in England and Wales: Year ending September 2020*. Gov.UK. Crown Copyright. https://www.ons.gov.uk/peoplepopulationandcommunity/crimeandjustice/bulletins/crimeinenglandandwales/yearendingseptember2020

United States Secret Service. (2020). *Secret service announces the creation of the cyber fraud task force*. https://www.secretservice.gov/newsroom/releases/2020/07/secret-service-announces-creation-cyber-fraud-task-force

Chapter 1

Cybersecurity is here to stay

Introduction

The very nature of the work you do – which can involve delving into the most sensitive, protected and personal areas of a person's life – means a need to protect all client data. Confidentiality and safeguarding clients are among the first basic things learnt by all coaches, therapists, counsellors, psychologists, researchers and practitioners in care-giving roles. This chapter presents an honest view of how these factors fit into today's technological world and outlines the foundations of why every practitioner needs to learn to be cybersecure if they want to keep client data safe as well as client–practitioner interactions secure (whether written or spoken).

After reading this chapter you will have more awareness on

The home office

Including an understanding of what a home office and working from home actually mean today on both sides – for you as a practitioner and for your clients. While some readers may be employed by a corporation, many may be self-employed, working from a home set-up or a small office with equipment set up by themselves. Others may be working both in a corporation and a home office set-up.

Why cybersecurity is important?

Demonstrated through a discussion of the growing threat of cybercrime, highlighting the reasons why you need to self-educate on how to combat this.

Why the healthcare sector is a target?

Through an explanation of why occupations that fall under healthcare are targeted by cybercriminals, a trend that does not currently show any sign of abatement.

*

DOI: 10.4324/9781003184805-2

Terminology and your role

For simplification, the term "practitioners" is used throughout the book to group everyone this book is aimed at: coaches, therapists, psychologists, counsellors, researchers and other professionals handling confidential client data. This choice was made purely to have one term to cover all the readers. The term "client" is similarly used to group anyone practitioners work with.

Definitions of the term "cybersecurity" can vary, and often include references to protecting networks and devices. Overall, for the reader of this book, cybersecurity includes being able to detect, mitigate and stop vulnerabilities, risks or attacks on your devices, networks and data. It also covers knowing how to respond in the event of an attack occurring.

It is important to point out that, in today's world, it is unlikely that any practitioner has zero touch points to the cyberspace and works without any form of connected electronic device (computer, tablet, phone or other). This would require that you correspond with clients only through face-to-face communication, never on a phone or other electronic device, never over email and never over any communications software/apps. It would also mean you never store session notes, calendar entries or static data related to your clients on a computer, tablet, smartphone or other electronic device. Also, to be clear, data written offline on a device disconnected from a network does not make it "safe" from cybercriminals; it can still be taken if the device is stolen or when the device goes online again. As soon as you touch the cyberspace, you are open to the risks this book will lay out. The book further funnels all of this down, chapter-by-chapter, to the focus points relevant to the reader.

Other useful terminology to understand at this point is that cybercrime is often delineated into cyber enabled and cyber dependent. Cyber-dependent crimes are those that rely on electronic devices (both on the criminal and the victim side) and a network connection to execute the crime – at least initially (Europol, 2017). Ransomware (which will be covered later) is an example of a cyber-dependent crime. Cyber-enabled crimes are crimes executed via the cyberspace, but not fully reliant on it. An easy way to distinguish this is: could the crime be committed in another format offline (The Crown Prosecution Service [CPS], 2019)? For example, you can be scammed for money by someone talking to you face-to-face, or via some form of correspondence over a computer, the cyberspace just enables a new, escalated or alternative form of the scam.

These definitions prompt a very important reminder on cybersecurity for the audience of this book: practitioners have a responsibility to understand their role in reducing the "dependent" and "enabled" factors of these crimes through cybersecurity and their own awareness. As will be shown in Chapters 5–7, some cybercrimes rely on weak security, while others rely on a person falling victim to a story.

You are operating in occupations where the term "confidentiality" is one of the main foundations of working with a client. Ensuring this and protecting client information starts from the very first contact. Data should be understood as comprising anything related to a client, including all interactions. The bottom line is that the moment you handle, process or store data insecurely, which includes having a conversation insecurely, you leave a door open for a criminal or an opportunist – to obtain the data either through unauthorised access online or by physically stealing it offline.

Most accreditation bodies/associations practitioners are members of now include references to data security in their ethics codes and competency frameworks or other guidelines. However, these are often just references with limited interpretation of what is written. As a practical guide, this book, by applying the cybersecurity lens, gives the reader more insight into why these regulations are there – not only to protect clients but all of us. By incorporating practices to protect data, we also make our entire practice less vulnerable. This is vital because where practitioners work from the foundations of confidentiality and trust, criminals operate from the opposite side of the spectrum. Their strategies are built around finding vulnerabilities that will enable them to exploit victims, and the more sensitive the data, the more valuable it is.

With technology comes responsibility

Before the advent of computers, client data was vulnerable where it was, in the physical space where it was written or lay locked up in fireproof safes or cabinets, which meant that it could only be taken from that one place. Today, however, emails, calendar events and notes connecting a practitioner to a client are typically stored on devices that can be moved around and connected online.

The ease with which we can store data and make it portable, along with the increasing vulnerabilities in the cyberspace, has likely been part of why there has been an increase in privacy and data protection laws over the last decades (Solove, 2007). The challenge is that the cyberspace today enables more entry points for criminals and more extraction points for them to take your data and listen in on your conversations.

An important point to make here is that a breach of privacy or data occurs when any type of record is taken. One online session overheard by a stranger, one exposed chat message thread or the breach of a calendar app and all its records, including the names and contact information of clients, is enough to threaten exposure of your clients and even bluff that more information is held. As will be highlighted through a real-life story coming up in this chapter, the fear of what might have been exposed can be enough to create emotional responses in clients. The breach of trust factor is significant.

All these points said, working online today is not only unavoidable but also enables practitioners to potentially provide more services, more efficiently than before. Storing client information electronically means it is available from anywhere at any time, and engaging in digital communication may improve outcomes dramatically for some clients, who would otherwise struggle to attend onsite (for either practical or health reasons). So, while the realities of cybercrime will be pulled into focus in this chapter, do not let this deter you; rather, the information is being provided to firmly show why cybersecurity is here to stay.

Another important point is that not all cyberthreats will target your clients' data. Some will be aimed at extracting money from you, through scams aimed at your business or you as the practitioner. These are also unfolded in this book, along with how to spot and mitigate them. Learning how to mitigate these threats is arguably just as important as protecting your client data, because cybercrime and fraud can cause long-lasting damage either financially or personally – to the extent that it can then have ripple effects on clients, leading to a situation where the practitioner either needs to discontinue or close their practice.

A final note on the important role you play in this journey. When working with clients, human behaviour and cognition may often be important factors in choices and outcomes for them. Although cybersecurity relies on technology and tools, human factors play a crucial role there too, particularly against criminals who continuously will look for a way in, and do not have any boundaries. By understanding the why, what and how and starting to implement some good practices along with reading these chapters, you minimise your own vulnerability as well as the weaknesses in your technology set-up.

In summary, it is through taking an active part in learning about cybercrime, understanding how to spot red flags as well as setting up security tools, that you enable a holistic, more effective cybersecurity approach (Back & LaPrade, 2019). Through changing behaviours and practices you can also build further on what you learn in the future, and much of what you read here can also be adapted into your everyday, personal cybersecurity practices.

Why being fully offline is not actually a safer option

There is no silver-bullet solution to any of the cyberthreats or issues mentioned in this book, unfortunately. The reality is that if one source of income for a cybercriminal is closed off, they will explore a new modus operandi (MO), look for new ways in, find the next security flaw or vulnerable person to exploit. It can be tempting, then, to consider that taking an alternative route to cybersecurity is having a no digital, online footprint – or a reduced one.

The problem is, this doesn't work any longer either and would just reduce the client experience of being able to reach you digitally. Security expert Brian Krebs (2020b) has pointed out that the pride some people have had in how they have avoided using the internet and online accounts for anything that involves personal or financial data may be the type of pride that comes before a fall. In today's world, not having registered and gained control over your digital identity – where there are opportunities to do so – means someone else might do so for you. Gaining online access to government-related accounts, banking services, pensions, tax, credit, driver's licencing and other accounts with online access may not require a significant amount of information for a criminal if access has not been established before. Krebs describes the importance of planting "your virtual flag" – enabling online access where you can before someone else does (2020a, 2020b). Each area of a digital identity a criminal obtains access to can also enable them to move to the next.

Tip: Consider people around you, outside of the professional sphere. Do you have an elderly or vulnerable relative who has never banked online (and especially consider if they have told others of this)? It can be safer to set them up and put maximum security controls on that access and what can be done with that access, than keep them offline, where someone else might set up access in their place. Discuss with their bank to explore options. Similarly, ensure that they have set up any extra controls, such as multi-factor authentication (MFA), before a criminal or an opportunist does (Krebs, 2020b).

Threats to the home office set-up

Launching into the 2020s, it was impossible not to pause for a small reflection on a hundred years earlier. The 1920s had been a decade of economic boom and cultural change, thus earning the expression the "Roaring Twenties". The decade offered new freedoms to women, and many industries, such as transport, medicine and media, grew, expanded and started to thrive. Jazz and dance clubs dominated a thriving social scene. A century later, the 2020s started a little differently. Aeroplanes – which, in the 1920s, many people wanted to try and experience – were grounded and out of bounds. Our medical field was overrun by a pandemic, leading to lockdowns that flattened the social scene. During isolation due to COVID-19 restrictions, people turned inward. Reliance on online media (essentially any way of communicating online) became a necessity – via our now omnipresent internet, which is difficult to live without.

Online media and the internet became facilitators, among other things, for the following:

1. Social contact where physical contact was not possible
2. Purchase of goods and food
3. Work – enabling continuation of work for many from a home instead of an on-location office or other environment

All of this was possible and part of many people's lives pre-2020 and pre-pandemic. A new reliance and an accelerated, increased use of such possibilities occurred, however. The expanding use of the cyberspace means that many, including practitioners, will continue to have more online work opportunities post-pandemic. The changing times have, however, also drawn the interest of cybercriminals towards targeting people working from home. Many readers may have seen increased media coverage of the weaknesses of a home office set-up or online media tools during this period (Patterson, 2021). More on all of this will be unpacked in this section to demonstrate some of the initial reasons a practitioner needs to become cyber aware and competent at their own cybersecurity.

First, let's look at what working from home (WFH) or a home office can look like, for both practitioner and client, before going deeper.

Practitioners may be

1.   Working from a home office or other personal practice space (operating alone or as part of a small business) they have set up themselves
2.   Offering online and/or onsite services
3.   Working as associates or employees of a company or institution (in a role linked to their professional field). Working onsite or a mix of onsite and via logging into the company's systems from a home office set-up
4.   Completing temporary/short-term contracts, executed online from a home office set-up, or onsite at the offices of companies/corporates they are hired to work for. (This may be as a consultant or contracted party for a particular work engagement.)
5.   Undertaking a mix of roles – personal practice and working as an associate or a consultant for companies (or any other combination)

It is important to note that whichever combination of the aforementioned you fall under, it will be rare to meet a practitioner who is never using a device, a network or an office space essentially under their own responsibility to secure. Two scenarios:

•   Where 3 or 4 applies to you and none of the others, evaluate still if you only use the devices of the companies on their premises and network. Often, practitioners will prepare or log in from their own home-based set-up
•   If you work for multiple companies, you may also still use your own devices (particularly if you are contracted) as well as your own home office space

Clients may

1.   Be seeking face-to-face, onsite services only
2.   Prefer an online practitioner to reduce travel time
3.   Seek a mixture of onsite and online support
4.   Simply have preferences not to meet at a practitioner's place of work due to safety or other concerns

5.   Want to work with a particular coach, counsellor or therapist recommended to them, but who is not within reasonable travel distance and therefore they require online services

The client view centres around finding the right practitioner and a session type that suits them in terms of format and availability. Although many clients will consider data security in terms of privacy laws where they have become aware of their rights over their own data (dependent on their location), they probably rarely consider the security of their data from a technological, cybersecurity point of view. This leaves the balance of responsibility and the motivation to ensure a cybersecure practice weighted towards the practitioner. How practitioners need to connect the dots between data laws, ethics and cybersecurity comes later on, in Chapter 8. For now, let's continue looking at where the practitioner is working.

The corporate influence

In this section, let's just look a bit closer at the WFH influence from the corporate space. As a practitioner, you may or may not have working contact with companies or the corporate world. Many of your clients do, however, and there is some wisdom to glean from this as one world can affect another. Examples:

- Clients now used to working online more may seek more online and remote services for themselves than before, after experiencing its convenience when working
- The fact that the pandemic was a driver for a greater focus on cybersecurity stems heavily from the corporate world going home to work

While, as already noted, some practitioners may not have felt a large shift in working practices, the society and systems we are under have very much shifted. Along with the increased WFH focus has come the increased focus of cybercriminals on attacking home offices (ECHO, 2020).

The corporate world was arguably anyway heading towards a more flexible working structure for employees. WFH and remote or virtual work (not having to go to an office) has been seen as "inevitable" (Li et al., 2020). Before the current WFH trend, a 2016 field study revealed that, on average, employees would give up to 8% of their salary to work from home (Mas & Pallais, 2017). A quick internet search today returns countless studies that took advantage of collecting data in 2020–2021; these show the different sides of people's impression of how WFH full time was actually experienced during the pandemic. On one side, some employees would like to continue working remotely and away from the buildings or offices of a place of work, feeling more productive at home (McKinsey, 2020). On the other side, novel health issues connected to working from home came up during the pandemic including reductions in physical and mental wellbeing from working in a new environment. That new environment being homes perhaps not intended before for work, often without typical workstation tools and with more distractions (other household members or children present), all fuelled by the intensity of speed of this evolution (Xiao et al., 2021).

The new WFH revolution occurred over a matter of weeks. There was little time to even consider how to adjust to a home working culture or the potential impact on personal health (Li et al., 2020). While academics and practitioners quickly responded by studying the best ways to support the workplace mindset shift and wellbeing needs (Oakman et al., 2020; Van Nieuwerburgh et al., 2021), it takes time for findings and support to filter through all layers of a company. The same has been the case for cybersecurity, which has come second to getting people operational in a home office space. Cyberattacks increased in the pandemic due to the lack of preparedness of many companies in readying a safe and secure home-office set up for staff (Furnell & Shah, 2020). Some companies are still catching up, which will be particularly important where they intend to continue to offer a blended home/office set-up for staff going forward (McKinsey, 2020). This means the increased interest of criminals on home networks will continue – think of the Eye of Sauron from *The Lord of the Rings*. The focus has tuned in, meaning everyone remains more vulnerable and there is no one ring to melt to stop it.

The practitioner's new view

For practitioners, working online from a home set-up or private practice has been common enough to have sparked significant research on the effectiveness and challenges of providing online counselling, therapy and coaching (Barak et al., 2009; Leibert et al., 2006; Berninger-Schäfer, 2018; Situmorang, 2020). Both the demand for online services and the effectiveness of it for some clients are not questioned. However, quite simply, working from a home set-up increases attack vectors and risks to data (Pranggono & Arabo, 2021). In cybersecurity, all the ways a cybercriminal can infiltrate are often called "attack vectors". The rest of this chapter will unfold why this is the case.

To be clear, all the cybersecurity weaknesses noted through this book have been around for some time. Even without the ever-increasing use of online technology to connect and provide services, without pandemics and without the WFM revolution of the early 2020s, the information in this book is simply long overdue. Even in 2006, the cyber issues related to the home worker were being raised as needing attention (Furnell, 2006). The volume of workers adapting to the new lifestyle during the pandemic has just increased attention from criminals. Targeting home offices and home networks has become more interesting now there are more targets. Weaknesses that were previously ignored or underexploited beforeare now targeted as ways into a home-office or even further into the corporations the home-worker is connected to (Furnell & Shah, 2020; Pranggono & Arabo, 2021). There is now more at stake from developing capabilities to exploit home offices and home networks. The WFH work culture has, in summary, led to an increase of capabilities and interest in exploiting attack vectors connected to home offices on the one hand, and a new urgency and impetus to tackle this phenomenon, on the other.

Reflecting back, you may recall news stories around more people working or studying from home on topics such as hacked accounts, poor home cybersecurity and breaches. Most readers will have also seen a news story about "Zoombombing". In fact, many conferencing software products were actually targeted by people trying to disrupt services or listen into calls. It wasn't just Zoom, however. "Zoombombing" was the catchword that stuck, now even having its own Wikipedia entry (Zoombombing, 2021). For a practitioner, there are more cyberthreats than those mentioned so far and in news stories you may have read. By enumerating the most high-risk ones for your practice, this book will help you focus on building your capabilities towards mitigating these alongside setting up a more cybersecure practice.

The increase in cyberthreats and fraud, already noted, needs to be met by increasing numbers of people learning to combat such threats and thus keeping the online space secure. Until now, most of you have been following guidelines from licencing bodies, associations, or accreditation bodies, but may not have connected this to how data cannot really be secure if the cyberspace around it is not secure. In the next sections, we will unfold a few other reasons why any person handling confidential data today needs to become more skilled, competent and confident in the cybersecurity space.

Activity

This book will unfold information alongside very simple, practical, applicable exercises, and here is a gentle exercise to get us started. First, find a new notebook or open a document on your PC to document your reflections as you go through this book. This will only take you a couple of minutes here and there, and if you are accredited, you can even check if you are able to re-use later elements of what you write as reflective continuing professional development (CPD).

On your first page, note down some reflections on the following:

- What you know about cybersecurity and fraud prevention today
- How you believe you embed what you know into your daily practice today

We will return to these reflections later.

Mark's case – Part 1

I thought I was invincible, but I became one of the people you read about.

Mark

Mark is tired; it is late, and it has been a really long day. After finishing some chores at home and having dinner with his family, he decides to check through his work emails as he is really behind answering them. He scrolls through a couple of them. As usual, he is very careful not to click on anything that doesn't look right – he has read enough alerts on clicking on links. His friend fell for one of those once, he recollects – put all his money into an online investment. He was lucky his bank called and asked him to double-check everything, because, of course, it was some scam. Mark would never do that. He knows if it is too good to be true, it usually is.

The phone rings; the number comes up on his phone as the tax authorities. He knows he hasn't opened all his post, and there was at least one letter from them. He feels guilty and considers not answering, but it must be serious if they are now chasing him by phone.

He answers. A nice lady explains she is phoning from the tax return team. He immediately apologies profusely in case he is late with something. He is just waiting for his accountant to come back from maternity leave. The nice lady confirms he owes some money, but she can help him if he can pay part or all of it today.

He explains his accountant is not available, and he doesn't know right now what he owes. The nice lady suggests that he pay a portion, say 300 pounds, and then the rest by end of the month if that would suit him. Even better, she is happy to sort the initial payment now if he has a credit card handy.

Mark feels relieved – even if he has to find another accountant, he will now have time to do that and not have to figure it out all by himself. He digs out his Mastercard and gives her all the information he is asked for. The nice lady processes everything, including the final codes from his SMS, which was just the last step, she explains, to confirm he was paying his bill. Mark shoots a quick email to his accountant to check if she will be back in time or if he will need to find someone else and goes to bed feeling reassured.

Activity

Read through the case again.
   In your reflective notes document or notebook, write down what you think happens next.
   You will be provided more of Mark's story in the next chapter.

Self cyber care

Many of us working today in cybersecurity started ground up, with some taking courses afterwards to upskill. That picture is changing. Taking the United Kingdom as an example, 18-year-olds are now opting to study cybersecurity at universities (Daniel, 2020), and the government annually recruits for its cyber apprenticeship scheme (Government Security Profession, 2021). Even younger people are being encouraged to be curious about the topic, helped by initiatives such as classroom tools for primary school children (Barefoot Computing, n.d.) and national codebreaking contests, groups and resources (National Cyber Security Centre ([NCSC], 2021).

While tomorrow we may be resourced, skilled and ready to combat cybercrime, today we are chasing to fill a huge gap that is growing. The internet has become omniscient in our lives, to the point that it is now seen as an emerging human right through its ability to enable sharing of information and freedom of speech (Shackelford, 2019). We take our use of it for granted, along with the acceleration of digitalisation, which has facilitated online working. Our reliance on the internet may mean we do not want to see that the digital infrastructure around us is "porous" and "brittle" (Taddeo, 2019, p. 1) and that with ongoing digitalisation there will come more opportunities to attack, and attack successfully (Taddeo, 2019).

It is good to consider, before filtering down to where we are responsible as practitioners, that cybersecurity and fraud pervade at all levels and in all countries. The World Economic Forum lists cybersecurity failure in the top ten global risks by likelihood (World Economic Forum, 2021). While the United States, the United Kingdom and India are the top three countries potentially facing particularly significant attacks (Specops Software, 2020), they happen everywhere. In 2020, Brazil's Superior Court was offline for more than a day and experienced disruption for a few weeks after being hit (Mari, 2020), and in 2021, a major telecom network in Belgium became the victim of a cyberattack, which affected private users and was connected to a subsequent sustained cyberattack on the government, also a user of the network (Montalbano, 2021).

Here are a few examples that illuminate further how criminals are not afraid of *who* they go after. In 2020, FireEye, one of the largest security firms in the world, revealed that tools they used to test the defences of other firms, had been hacked (Mandia, 2020). This cyber incident became perhaps the biggest cybersecurity story hitting mainstream media that year – that of Solar-Winds. Articles will continue to be written about this attack for some years, unravelling how criminals could gain access to government and business computer networks through breaching IT performance-monitoring software called "Orion", developed by SolarWinds (SolarWinds, 2021). Criminals had installed vulnerabilities in the software – ready for when anyone else installed the product. This attack reached around 18,000 of SolarWinds' Orion customers, including the US government and companies such as Fire-Eye (Paul, 2020). These examples illuminate that if governments, security and tech companies are not impervious, then it should be clear that no one is, at any level and in any country. The examples also reveal how cyberattacks often unfold, over a period of time, enabling a patient (and painful) extraction of information. Some organised cybercrime groups are though starting to execute more quickly (Paganini, 2021).

Allianz produces a yearly business risk barometer report. While in previous years cyber risk had been a rising top priority for many companies, the impact and disruption of the pandemic and business disruption became focal points in 2021 (Allianz Global Corporate & Speciality, 2021). Businesses likely were forced to redirect resources towards enabling business continuity, working in new ways and navigating the economic downturn that can emerge at such times. Cyber risks themselves did not go away, however. As noted already, businesses adapted, so did cybercriminals. From their worldview, cybercriminals also need to make a living; when the landscape changes, it closes some opportunities and revenue streams and opens others. For example, in the last quarter of 2020, the growth in e-commerce potentially enabled fraudsters to gain, on average, 70% more per fraudulent purchase compared with that of the year before (Sift, 2020), the bounty coming from the increase in online traffic and sales from the environment of the COVID-19 pandemic. While shop doors were closed, criminals found new techniques to go under the detection radars of merchants, cards issuers and banks to take advantage of increased online transaction levels (Sift, 2020).

Cyber skills and business owners

A UK cybersecurity labour market survey in 2021 showed that 50% of all UK businesses have a gap in basic cybersecurity-related skills (DCMS, 2021), and this was also an increase of 2% on the figure from the year before (DCMS, 2020). Statistics like this can be found in any country along with other details. The Australian Computer Society, for example, stated that small businesses made up more than 97% of all businesses in 2019 in Australia, with 62% of those belonging to sole traders and 27% having 1–4 staff (Braue, 2019). Sole traders, the self-employed and small businesses do not typically have extra resources or a business size that can justify an IT department, or staff who can set up and maintain extensive cybersecurity. This also means that they do not have experts to set up secure defences and are unable to cope if a cyber incident occurs (Gafni & Pavel, 2019).

Additionally, while cybercriminals have continued to hone their abilities to conduct cyberattacks, many practitioners have spent the last years grappling with data and privacy legislation purely from a regulatory point of view. Little targeted information has been provided on the digital, practical side of keeping data safe in a cyber world. This means that while many practitioners are able to say that they apply the legislation, they may be without the competences to actually keep their practice and their client data confidential and safe from breaches.

If you have worked for yourself for a long time and not for a corporation, your only sources of information on computers and cybersecurity may have been what you have seen in the media, learnt from others or educated yourself on. When you are working at a corporation or a business, there are often yearly mandatory training programmes on a variety of topics aimed at keeping you, the company you work for or its customers safe. Osterman Research Inc (2019) estimates the return on investment (ROI) for even a small organisation (50 people up) in security awareness training as 69%. ROI here can be understood as a return on preventing financial loss. The figures indicate training may be effective. Some companies also see cyber training as part of overarching corporate or social sustainability strategies (Shackelford, 2019). However, even with company-level training, setting up security at home is different and reliant on the abilities you have and security tools you select.

This is where this book comes in. For the smaller practice or for independent practitioners performing all IT administration and technical set-ups yourself, this book will help to supplement for a lack of cyber training as well as build cybersecurity awareness. For larger practices with cyber support or IT support, the book can still be provided to employees to make them more aware of which risks surround them, how to spot red flags and how to react if something happens.

Chapters 2–4 will help you build layers of defence around your data and practice through topics such as secure networks, devices and software usage. The information will complement any training or learning you undertake yourself, and it also provides an overview of many of the risks directly applicable to the professions this book is aimed at, enabling a streamlining of information to what you need practically to secure your practice and client data. Allowing you, as you read to immediately use and apply many of the principles suggested.

Healthcare as a target

As many practitioners will be working in the healthcare space, this section focuses on it. However, many may also have roles in educational establishments – teaching or training others or performing research. It is therefore worth mentioning that the education sector is also widely targeted. This is why many educational establishments have strict cybersecurity policies as well as ethics guidelines for research, data storage and software use. Both healthcare and education are sectors where there is something to lose – records that, if revealed or destroyed, can impact the person they pertain to. What would happen if your education records were completely deleted? What would happen if your medical files are gone or revealed to the public? As will be unfolded in this section, data is a valuable commodity, and attacks on healthcare have been climbing along with the exposure of records and data breaches as a result (Seh et al., 2020). More later on the financial statistics.

So far it was highlighted that cybersecurity is often challenging for the self-employed and for small businesses. However, let's now be clear that this book will help change that view and also that cybersecurity has not necessarily been easier for medium-sized or larger therapist, counselling or coaching services to navigate either. The attacks on them are also more likely to reach the headlines due to the scale of impact. Those stories provide some good case studies of cyber-attacks on practitioners.

In the United States, one of the largest breaches of mental health records so far occurred in 2020, exposing a little over 295,000 patient records (Alder, 2020). Breaches like this are not new. In 2015, a data breach of around 11,000 patients at a Texas mental health facility was notified. In the investigation afterwards, it was discovered that an authorised user may have gained access to the records as early as 2012 (Alder, 2015). In Australia, Anglicare in Sydney fell victim to a cyber-attack in October 2020. Among other things, Anglicare provides mental health services and counselling. The breach was reported in the Australian media as a ransomware attack (Malone, 2020). The company itself did not appear to confirm the attack method but did state that it had strengthened its security, in statements about the incident on its website (Anglicare, 2020). In March 2022, Scottish mental health charity, SAMH, fell victim to a ransomware attack where attackers have claimed to have exfiltrated data.

Ransomware is a threat that has become more complex for healthcare in the last years and will be covered in Chapter 5 in more detail. In brief, it involves hackers infiltrating a company, often subsequently blocking the company from its own data or keeping a copy until a ransom is paid. The victim is threatened with deletion or exposure of the data if the ransom is not received by a deadline. One of the most vivid ransomware stories to read about is that of Vastaamo. Vastaamo is a Finland-based company running therapy centres across the country. The attack was revealed to the public in 2020 after it led to a significant data breach which is well depicted in some very emotive write ups by *Wired* on the aftermaths of patients exposed by this particular cyberattack (Ralston, 2020, 2021).

The story had great impact throughout the country; and hit the international press. Personal data and therapy notes were among the data stolen on around 37,000 patients. The shock within Finland at the lack of cybersecurity around sensitive data even led to legislative change around a person's ability to change their social security number in certain circumstances, such as being a victim of hacking (Helsinki Times, 2020). Ralston, in his articles for *Wired* (2020, 2021), provides accounts of some of the patients the attackers subsequently tried to blackmail individually, and how this affected them. He also quotes a Finnish cybersecurity research officer explaining how the case highlights the explosivity of sensitive medical records (Ralston, 2020).

The investigations afterwards revealed signs of cybersecurity negligence at Vastaamo and that the company was initially likely breached in November 2018 and March 2019. It was only in October 2020, however, that the situation came to light, expounding the media outcry. The gaps between when a company is first breached and when the company notices it, can indicate both a lack of controls at the company and the sophistication of the attack. Other reasons the Vastaamo case hit the media in style were that it was a ransomware attack, and when the company did not pay the ransom demanded by the hackers, things exploded. The hackers, determined not to back down, began to publish some of the data they had obtained, including that of well-known figures in society. They also started contacting the patients, blackmailing them for money under threat of having the notes of their private therapy sessions made public (Kleinman, 2020; Ralston, 2020).

Vastaamo is also a good example of how far the impact of a cyberattack can extend. In addition to the data exposure and impact on clients, the company ended up filing for bankruptcy, citing being ruined by the costs and uncertainty connected to the cyberattack and its aftermath (Scroxton, 2021). Damages for the breaches may still also have to be paid out (Yle, 2021). Through this book, you will be reminded periodically that most cyber risks applicable to practitioners can similarly lead to potential financial and reputation loss and thus similar outcomes. This is not to frighten you as reader, however. Remember that there were indications of security negligence in the Vastaamo case (Ralston, 2020). With the defences built up through these chapters and knowing how to react, each reader will be starting in another place when it comes to integrity. Companies do survive cyber incidents! However, in a case such as the one at Vastaamo, the breach of trust around the company's handling of sensitive data was likely insurmountable (Scroxton, 2021), especially once the details were made very visible in the media.

Stories about breaches of the self-employed practitioner and smaller practices are less likely to hit the media – not so much because they would be less emotional or less newsworthy, but rather because the media is not short of eye-catching stories pertaining to cyber incidents and breaches at larger healthcare institutions. These headlines have included a homicide case being opened after a death was initially seen as related to a cyberattack on a hospital in Germany (Tidy, 2020). Although this case was later closed, another case is continuing in court, in which a baby may have died due to monitoring systems not being available during a ransomware attack (Vaas, 2021).

In 2020, one cyberattack alone in the United States is thought to have led to the compromise of at least 10 million medical records, from a total 29 million healthcare records potentially breached over the same year (Alder, 2021). Again, don't think attacks on healthcare only occur in larger countries, by way of an example – in May 2021 alone, the healthcare sectors in Ireland and New Zealand were widely attacked (Greig, 2021).

Cyber care is for life

Lessons from the last section include the need to implement cybersecurity to fix and learn from issues, and improve on an ongoing, continuous basis. The Finnish and Texas cases, mentioned earlier, highlight how attention to fixing security weaknesses when the first breaches occurred may have prevented the latter outcomes. Another example of this that may encourage you to see how ongoing cybersecurity due diligence is necessary is one of the most written about cyberattacks that also affected the healthcare industry. This occurred in 2017. It was named WannaCry and had an impact on around 150 countries and approximately 300,000 devices (Akbanov et al., 2019). It has been written about extensively – partly due to the fact that the weakness was not remediated after the attack. This led to another large attack, not too long after, that targeted the same weakness, and was named NotPetya (Shackelford, 2019). WannaCry is also written about frequently, as the sophistication of the malware behind it is such that the malware has been used over and over again, impacting tens of thousands of healthcare institutions. Its inadequate mitigation means it is still being applied today (Forni, 2020; Berger, 2021).

Repetition is a theme through all cybercrime. Criminals will continue to exploit weaknesses and vulnerabilities until they are remediated. Methods that prove lucrative are extended, and go into a new MO to fit a new victim audience or to adjust around hurdles put in their path. Repetition also follows into scams. "Scampreneurs" (Button et al., 2009, p. 5) will use both open and illicit sources of information, including lists of people who have been a victim of a scam before – and end up on so-called sucker lists (Peachey, 2020).

As a practice owner, you will be directly targeted by scams that tune into your needs and vulnerabilities as a practice owner. The book will cover some of these scenarios and empower you towards creating life-long cyber-care practices, thus helping you protect your practice and client data from being exploited through the use of products that are not secure, vulnerable networks and unprotected devices and also from scammers. Cybersecurity is also not all about technology either. Much of this journey will be about making you more robust against the human errors, as these are also taken advantage of, along with security vulnerabilities and lapses, by criminals chasing your lucrative client data (Seh et al., 2020) and your bank balance.

Statistics were promised earlier. Exposed patient/client records have been reported as being sold on the darknet for up to US$1,000 or more (CBS News, 2019), whereas credit card numbers can sell for, in comparison, a lowly US$5 to 110 (Stack, 2017). A small disclaimer: as with any statistics, there is some variation in the prices reported, and the higher prices are linked to cases where the data record is more complete. For example, a complete medical record will fetch more than 'only' a social security number (CBS News, 2019).

Healthcare has lost billions to cyber-attacks, and criminals have been well-tuned to this sector for some time. One journalist even asked in 2016 whether healthcare hacking had become an epidemic (Akpan, 2016). In February 2021, the French president, Emmanuel Macron, announced a 1 billion Euro programme to combat cybercrime after 500,000 patient records were leaked in France in a cyber-attack (France24, 2021). During that exact same month, a cybersecurity resilience focused firm, IT Governance (Irwin, 2021), estimated that 2.3 billion records had been compromised globally. They noted the top three breached sectors as healthcare and health science, education and the public sector (Irwin, 2021).

Criminals, very simply, target healthcare because they can. There are vulnerabilities they are capable of exploiting; moreover, many of their victims will pay a ransom, knowing that the consequences of data being exposed can be very severe for the individuals the data pertains to. As mentioned earlier, after the Vastaamo attack, when the hackers did not get the payment they demanded from the company, they turned to blackmailing the individual clients since they had their full contact information as well as material from their sessions. One of these individuals, who was interviewed by *Wired* (Ralston, 2020), expressed how this left him feeling suicidal but also fearful of the legacy of it all for his family. Another had been a teenager when in therapy and was afraid of what the material in his session notes would mean for his future, if exposed (Ralston, 2021). The BBC also reported one Vastaamo client's description of the feeling of being blackmailed and his anxiety and fear over the things he had shared with his therapist being revealed. He was simply not ready for them to be known but was also not in a position to pay a ransom (Kleinman, 2020).

For you as practitioner – no matter the size of your practice or the sector you see it falling under – you can see the picture being painted in this section. Your data fits into this sensitive, lucrative, category. This coupled with the increasing focus of criminals on exploiting a home set-up and the digitisation of services, the purpose of this book should be becoming clearer. Cybercriminals are fully aware of what having access to your client records or conversations can earn them. They also know which buttons to press to scam you as well. All of this we will unpack in more detail.

It is important that we take a minute to reframe before moving to the conclusion of this chapter. Despite the statistics, cases and data so far, you can and should see this journey as a new venture. Your rucksack is empty, ready to be filled with resources. From Chapter 2 onwards, you will be able to pick those up and carry them with you. This book will not only inform you about how to activate different practices to protect yourself from vulnerabilities, but will also teach you in a conceptual, factual and reflective way, which will enable you to spot red flags and abnormalities yourself going forward. After you have read this book, it might stay on the shelf as something to turn to if something comes up, or to refresh or use the checklists at the end, but you will also be enabled and active in your own cybersecurity.

After putting into place solid foundations, you are less likely to be someone who ignores the first signs of a breach, unlike those in some of the cases given so far. You will also, going forward, better understand media reports on new threats in the future, and you will know what to do in the event anything happens.

Activity

Take out your reflective notes or open the document you are writing in. Re-read what you wrote in the first activity on what you know about cybersecurity and how you embed it into your practice today.

- Is there anything you want to add to your previous notes now?
- Note any questions that have started to come up. Later, you can check back if they are answered

- What has changed in your thinking, and what do you currently feel actioned to do?
- Note (at least) three positive things you believe you are going to get out of the rest of this book

Summary

The ethical codes, guidelines, legislation practitioners follow often clarify a need to keep data safe, and this chapter has presented elements of the "why" behind this and the connection to cybersecurity.

Areas covered included the following:

- The reasons practitioners need to upskill to protect their data and practice from cyber-enabled crime
- Clarity on the fact that practitioners operate with particularly sensitive data, which makes them a lucrative target
- Examples highlighting what can be lost due to cybercrime and the impact on clients
- How setting up good cybersecurity at home is required in order to keep a practice and its data (including conversations) secure

The media, banks, governments and others warn us about cyberattacks and cyber-enabled fraud regularly, but the connection into the practitioner's world may not always be clear. Chapter 2 is the first of three chapters looking at basic information on how to keep interactions and data secure from a practical perspective. It starts with the minimal basics, and the other chapters build from there, as you evolve into your own cyber specialist.

Working in professions where it is essential to keep everything between a practitioner and client confidential and safe, this book's information will build to enable you to achieve the data security standards you need to, and may be obliged to achieve, from ethical, data privacy and legal perspectives.

Self-cyber care is also about learning to spot the red flags of cybercrime and financial crime, and this book will later unfold some of the top threats. Everything together enables a new, greater understanding of the threats out there, the media stories, as well as "what" data legislation and ethics codes really are there for.

References

Akbanov, M., Vassilakis, V. G., & Logothetis, M. D. (2019). WannaCry ransomware: Analysis of infection, persistence, recovery. Prevention and propagation mechanisms. *Journal of Telecommunications & Information Technology*, *1*, 113–124. https://doi.org/10.26636/jtit.2019.130218

Akpan, N. (2016, March 23). *Has health care hacking become an epidemic*. PBS News. https://www.pbs.org/newshour/science/has-health-care-hacking-become-an-epidemic

Alder, S. (2015, October 26). *Hack discovered by emergence health network: 11K records exposed*. HIPPA Journal. https://www.hipaajournal.com/hack-discovered-by-emergence-health-network-11k-records-exposed/

Alder, S. (2020, December 1). *More than 295k patients impacted by cyberattack on AspenPointe*. HIPPA Journal. https://www.hipaajournal.com/more-than-295k-patients-impacted-by-cyberattack-on-aspenpointe/

Alder, S. (2021, January 19). *Healthcare data breach report: 25% increase in breaches in 2020*. HIPPA Journal. https://www.hipaajournal.com/2020-healthcare-data-breach-report-us/

Allianz Global Corporate & Specialty. (2021). *10th allianz risk barometer 2021*. https://www.agcs.allianz.com/news-and-insights/reports/allianz-risk-barometer.html

Anglicare. (2020, September 19). *Statement from Anglicare Sydney*. https://www.anglicare.org.au/about-us/media-releases/statement-from-anglicare-sydney-19-september-2020/

Back, S., & LaPrade, J. (2019). The future of cybercrime prevention strategies: Human factors and a holistic approach to cyber intelligence. *International Journal of Cybersecurity Intelligence & Cybercrime, 2*(2), 1–4. https://www.doi.org/10.52306/02020119KDHZ8339

Barak, A., Hen, L., Boniel-Nissim, M., & Shapira, N. (2009). A comprehensive review and a meta-analysis of the effectiveness of internet-based psychotherapeutic interventions. *Journal of Technology in Human Services, 26*, 109–160. https://doi.org/10.1080/15228830802094429

Barefoot Computing. (n.d.). *Be cybersmart*. https://www.barefootcomputing.org/cyber

Berger, M. (2021, March 2). Is wannacry still a threat? *Cybel Angel*. https://cybelangel.com/blog/wannacry-still-a-threat/

Berninger-Schäfer, E. (2018). *Online-coaching*. Springer.

Button, M., Lewis, C., & Tapley, J. (2009). *Fraud typologies and the victims of fraud: Literature review*. National Fraud Authority. https://assets.publishing.service.gov.uk/government/uploads/system/uploads/attachment_data/file/118469/fraud-typologies.pdf

Braue, D. (2019, November 28). *Can small business beat cyber skills crunch?* Australian Computer Society. https://ia.acs.org.au/article/2019/can-small-businesses-beat-cyber-skills-crunch-.html

CBS News. (2019, February 14). *Hackers are stealing millions of medical records – and selling them on the dark web*. CBS News. https://www.cbsnews.com/news/hackers-steal-medical-records-sell-them-on-dark-web/

The Crown Prosecution Service. (2019). *Cybercrime – prosecution guidance*. Crown Copyright. https://www.cps.gov.uk/legal-guidance/cybercrime-prosecution-guidance

Daniel, E. (2020, May 1). *UK government launches online cybersecurity courses for teenagers*. Verdict. https://www.verdict.co.uk/business/cybersecurity/online-cybersecurity-courses/

Department for Digital, Culture, Media and Sport (DCMS). (2020). *Cyber security skills in the UK labour market 2020*. Gov.UK. Crown Copyright. https://www.gov.uk/government/publications/cyber-security-skills-in-the-uk-labour-market-2020

Department for Digital, Culture, Media and Sport (DCMS). (2021). *Cyber security skills in the UK labour market 2021*. Gov.UK. Crown Copyright. https://www.gov.uk/government/publications/cyber-security-skills-in-the-uk-labour-market-2021

European network of Cyber security centres and competence Hub for innovation and Operations (ECHO). (2020, April 8). *The COVID-19 hackers mind-set*. ECHO White Paper no. 1. https://echonetwork.eu/wp-content/uploads/2020/04/20200408-ECHO-WhitePaper-Hackers-Mindset-FINAL.pdf

Europol. (2017). *Cyber dependent crime.* https://www.europol.europa.eu/iocta/2017/CYBER-DEPENDENT_CRIME.html

Forni, I. (2020, May 13). WannaCry 3 years later, could it happen again? *EclecticIQ.* https://blog.eclecticiq.com/wannacry-3-years-later-could-it-happen-again

France24. (2021, February 25). *France investigates leak of almost 500,000 medical records, including HIV and fertility status.* France24. https://www.france24.com/en/europe/20210225-france-investigates-massive-leak-of-medical-records

Furnell, S. (2006). Securing the home worker. *Network Security, 11,* 6–12. https://doi.org/10.1016/S1353-4858(06)70451-2

Furnell, S., & Shah, J. N. (2020). Home working and cyber security – an outbreak of unpreparedness? *Computer Fraud & Security, 8,* 6–12. https://doi.org/10.1016/S1361-3723(20)30084-1

Gafni, G., & Pavel, T. (2019). The invisible hole of information on SMB's cybersecurity. *Online Journal of Applied Knowledge Management (OJAKM), 7*(1), 14–26.

Government Security Profession. (2021, April 21). *Applications for the 2021 cyber apprentice scheme in government security are now open.* Crown Copyright. https://securityprofession.blog.gov.uk/2021/04/21/applications-for-the-2021-cyber-apprentice-scheme-in-government-security-are-now-open/

Greig, J. (2021, May 20). *Healthcare organizations in Ireland, New Zealand and Canada facing intrusions and ransomware attacks.* ZDnet. https://www.zdnet.com/article/healthcare-organizations-in-ireland-new-zealand-and-canada-facing-intrusions-and-ransomware-attacks/

Greig, J. (2022, March 22). *Ransomware group attacks Scottish mental health charity.* The Record.https://therecord.media/ransomware-group-attacks-scottish-mental-health-charity/

Helsinki Times. (2020, November 13). *Finland to make changing social security number easier for hacking victims.* Helsinki Times. https://www.helsinkitimes.fi/finland/finland-news/domestic/18312-finland-to-make-changing-social-security-number-easier-for-hacking-victims.html

Irwin, L. (2021, March 1). *List of data breaches and cyber attacks in February 2021 – 2.3 billion records breached.* IT Governance. https://www.itgovernance.co.uk/blog/list-of-data-breaches-and-cyber-attacks-in-february-2021-2-3-billion-records-breached

Kleinman, Z. (2020, October 26). *Therapy patients blackmailed for cash after clinic data breach.* BBC News. https://www.bbc.com/news/technology-54692120

Krebs, B. (2020a, June 19). *Turn on MFA before crooks do it for you.* Krebs on Security. https://krebsonsecurity.com/2020/06/turn-on-mfa-before-crooks-do-it-for-you/

Krebs, B. (2020b, August 12). *Why and where you should plant your flag.* Krebs on Security. https://krebsonsecurity.com/2020/08/why-where-you-should-you-plant-your-flag/

Leibert, T., Archer, J., Munson, J., & York, G. (2006). An exploratory study of client perceptions of internet counseling and the therapeutic alliance. *Journal of Mental Health Counseling, 28*(1), 69–83. https://doi.org/10.17744/mehc.28.1.f0h37djrw89nv6vb

Li, J., Ghosh, R., & Nachmias, S. (2020). In a time of COVID-19 pandemic, stay healthy, connected, productive, and learning: Words from the editorial team of HRDI. *Human Resource Development International, 23*(3), 199–207. https://doi.org/10.1080/13678868.2020.1752493

Malone, U. (2020, September 19). *Anglicare Sydney being held to ransom over sensitive data stolen from computer system.* ABC News.https://www.abc.net.au/news/2020-09-19/anglicare-sydney-victim-of-cyber-security-breach-involving-data/12681510

Mandia, K. (2020, December 8). FireEye shares details of recent cyber attack, actions to protect community. *Fire Eye*. https://www.fireeye.com/blog/products-and-services /2020/12/fireeye-shares-details-of-recent-cyber-attack-actions-to-protect-community. html

Mari, A. (2020, November 6). *Brazilian superior electoral court hit by major cyberattack*. ZDNet. https://www.zdnet.com/article/brazilian-superior-electoral-court-hit-by -major-cyberattack/

Mas, A., & Pallais, A. (2017). Valuing alternative work arrangements. *American Economic Review, 107*(12), 3722–3759. https://doi.org/10.1257/aer.20161500

McKinsey Global Internet. (2020, September 23). *What 800 executives envision for the post pandemic workforce*. https://www.mckinsey.com/featured-insights/future-of-work /what-800-executives-envision-for-the-postpandemic-workforce

Montalbano, E. (2021, May 6). *Massive DDoS attack disrupts Belgium parliament*. Threat Post. https://threatpost.com/ddos-disrupts-belgium/165911/

National Cyber Security Centre. (2021, February 11). *Thousands of girls take on code-breaking puzzles in bid to win UK cybersecurity crown*. Crown Copyright. https://www .ncsc.gov.uk/news/girls-take-on-codebreaking-puzzles

Oakman, J., Kinsman, N., Stuckey, R., Graham, M., & Weale, V. (2020). A rapid review of mental and physical health effects of working at home: How do we optimise health? *BMC Public Health, 20*, 1825. https://doi.org/10.1186/s12889-020-09875-z

Osterman Research. (2019, August 19). *The ROI of security awareness training – white paper*. https://ostermanresearch.com/2019/08/19/orwp_0313/

Paganini, P. (2021, December 8). *Emotet directly drops Cobalt Strike beacons without intermediate Trojans*. Security Affairs. https://securityaffairs.co/wordpress/125384 /cyber-crime/emotet-cobalt-strike.html

Patterson, D. (2021, May 19). *Cybercrime is thriving during the pandemic, driven by surge in phishing and ransomware*. CBS News. https://www.cbsnews.com/news /ransomware-phishing-cybercrime-pandemic/

Paul, K. (2020, December 15). What you need to know about the biggest hack of the US government in years. *The Guardian*. https://www.theguardian.com/technology/2020 /dec/15/orion-hack-solar-winds-explained-us-treasury-commerce-department

Peachey, K. (2020, December 23). *Brazen fraudsters offer crime subscription service*. BBC News. https://www.bbc.com/news/business-55424091

Pranggono, B., & Arabo, A. (2021). COVID-19 pandemic cybersecurity issues. *Internet Technology Letters*. https://doi.org/10.1002/itl2.247

Ralston, W. (2020, December 9). *A dying man, a therapist and the ransom raid that shook the world*. Wired. https://www.wired.co.uk/article/finland-mental-health-data-breach-vastaamo

Ralston, W. (2021, May 4). *They told their therapists everything: Hackers leaked it all*. Wired. https://www.wired.co.uk/article/finland-mental-health-data-breach-vastaamo

Scroxton, A. (2021, February 11). *Hacked Finnish therapy business collapses*. Computer-Weekly.com. https://www.computerweekly.com/news/252496227/Hacked-Finnish-therapy-business-collapses

Seh, A. H., Zarour, M., Alenezi, M., Sarkar, A. K., Agrawal, A., Kumar, R., & Kahn, A. K. (2020). Healthcare data breaches: Insights and implications. *Healthcare, 8*(2). https://doi.org/10.3390/healthcare8020133

Shackelford, S. J. (2019). Should cybersecurity be a human right? Exploring the "shared responsibility" of cyber peace (2017). *Stanford Journal of International Law No.*

2019, *Kelley School of Business Research Paper No. 17–55*. http://doi.org/10.2139
/ssrn.3005062

Sift. (2020). *Q4 2020 digital trust & safety index: Holiday fraud and the shifting state of e-commerce*. https://resources.sift.com/ebook/digital-trust-safety-index-holiday-fraud-shifting-ecommerce/

Situmorang, D. D. B. (2020). Online/cyber counseling services in the COVID-19 outbreak: Are they really new? *Journal of Pastoral Care & Counseling, 74*(3), 166–174. https://doi.org/10.1177/1542305020948170

SolarWinds. (2021). *SolarWinds security advisory*. https://www.solarwinds.com/sa-overview/securityadvisory#anchor1

Solove, D. J. (2007). The new vulnerability: Data security and personal information. In A. Chander, L. Gelman, & M. J. Radin (Eds.), *Securing privacy in the Internet age* (pp. 1–18). Palo Alto, CA: Stanford University Press.

Specops Software. (2020, July 13). *The countries experiencing the most "significant" cyber-attacks*. https://specopssoft.com/blog/countries-experiencing-significant-cyber-attacks/

Stack, B. (2017, September 6). Here's how much your personal information is selling for on the dark web. *Experian*. https://www.experian.com/blogs/ask-experian/heres-how-much-your-personal-information-is-selling-for-on-the-dark-web/

Taddeo, M. (2019). Is cybersecurity a public good? *Minds & Machines, 29*, 349–354. https://doi.org/10.1007/s11023-019-09507-5

Tidy, J. (2020, September 18). Police launch homicide inquiry after German hospital hack. *BBC News*. https://www.bbc.co.uk/news/technology-54204356

Vaas, L. (2021, September 30). *Baby's death alleged to be linked to ransomware*. Threat Post. https://threatpost.com/babys-death-linked-ransomware/175232/

Van Nieuwerburgh, C., Barr, M., Fouracres, A. J. S., Moin, T., Brown, C., Holden, C., Lucey, C., & Thomas, P. (2021). Experience of positive psychology coaching while working from home during the COVID-19 pandemic: An interpretative phenomeno-logical analysis. *Coaching: An International Journal of Theory, Research and Practice*. https://doi.org/10.1080/17521882.2021.1897637

World Economic Forum. (2021). *The global risks report 2021* (16th ed.). https://www3.weforum.org/docs/WEF_The_Global_Risks_Report_2021.pdf

Xiao, Y., Becerik-Gerber, B., Lucas, G., & Roll, S. C. (2021). Impacts of working from home during COVID-19 pandemic on physical and mental well-being of office work-station users. *Journal of Occupational and Environmental Medicine, 63*(3), 181–190. https://doi.org/10.1097/JOM.0000000000002097

Yle. (2021, February 2). *Hacked psychotherapy centre Vastaamo files for bankruptcy*. https://yle.fi/uutiset/osasto/news/hacked_psychotherapy_centre_vastaamo_files_for_bankruptcy/11785891

Zoombombing. (2021, December 3). *In Wikipedia*. https://en.wikipedia.org/wiki/Zoombombing

Chapter 2

Securing PCs and other devices

As promised, we are starting with the very basics. This chapter begins with the technological basics of protecting devices. This provides the foundation for the chapters that follow, which will graduate into areas that may be newer to you and will also include specific threats and the important role people play in ensuring good cybersecurity.

The gentle starting point is security software, as it would be hard to find someone who has no knowledge of this area. Most of you will, as a minimum, be aware of the need to have an "anti-virus" product installed on your computer. The chapter will go deeper into what to look for in security products and how to select them for mobile devices as well as computers.

Activity

Note your answers to these questions in your reflective notes:

Do you know which anti-virus/security software product is installed on your computer?
Is it the best-possible protection for your computer?
How often does it scan your computer?
What exactly does it protect you from?
Are you fully aware that you need to protect all your electronic devices?

DOI: 10.4324/9781003184805-3

The chapter will build the following:

Awareness

of the importance of having security software running on your devices

Understanding

of why data security goes beyond your computer to any electronic device you use

of how to research for the best products yourself

Improved ethical practices

around the choices you make and your responsibility to protect the devices you use with updated, reliable technology

---

A little time spent now ensuring your data is safely inside your fortress will mean your troops have a better chance of keeping it there if you are attacked.

---

*

Computer security software

Security software can help prevent real-time threats through detection and, where possible, mitigation of them. It enables a device to be protected from threats known to the product you use. We start with this, before moving on to other ways to protect devices, and we start with PCs. Note that the term "security software" is used here interchangeably with "anti-virus software" – as most products have moved on to perform more than just anti-virus protection today. When these products first came about, they were often called "anti-virus software", and many products as well as users still use this term.

Many people use a security software product they have used for many years and have become comfortable with, moving it from one PC to the next. Others make use of the "offers" that pop up when you get the PC out of the box and start it up. Both of these methods of protecting a device seem intuitive and simple. Unfortunately, using the same product for years without re-evaluating it, or using the product that came as a trial on your new PC, is the easy option. The security software you have used for many years may feel easy to use through its familiarity, but it may no longer be the leading choice to protect your PC. The security software a PC manufacturer pre-loads into its computers might be a product they consider the best out there, but it might also just be a product they have a deal with to add as a trial to all new computers. It is important to review the functionality (and pricing) of alternatives.

This chapter will guide you on how to make informed security software choices for the devices you have. Cybercriminals are constantly trying to find new vulnerabilities and ways in. It takes a strong, well-driven product to keep up, meaning that the best product one day may be overtaken by another tomorrow. Some products go from strength to strength, while others do not, this is why the book will not recommend any particular brands or security software companies. Instead the advice in the next sections will empower you to keep up with the changing threat landscape and evolution of products by regularly researching the product you use. It will also inform you of the importance of being more precisely aware of what it is protecting you against.

You will also be guided through the relevance of being able to actively use your security software and finding a product you understand and feel comfortable navigating. There may be a product that might protect you more or suit you better that you haven't tried yet. It might even be cheaper and easier to use than the ones you have used before. By the end of the chapter, you will learn how to select the one most appropriate for your needs, meaning from now, and going forward, you will have the skills to do so yourself.

Some operating systems (OSs) offer their own anti-virus today without extra charge. Microsoft offers Windows Defender, for example. The chapter will provide thoughts for reflection around the use of free security products. This will be touched upon so that you may make informed choices on whether they are adequate for your needs.

PC security software – moving beyond the status quo

As noted, just because your computer came with product X, or just because you have been using product Y for ten years with no problems, does not mean you need not look further. You should not continue using product Y for another decade without doing a review. As part of the action steps in this chapter, you will perform a review as you read. Going forward, the best time to re-review your products is the month before their renewal. Or, if you are using a free product, periodically verify whether what it is covering is still sufficient for you.

When reviewing and evaluating security products, the following resources can be used:

1. security/technology review websites
2. websites of the products
3. articles on the strengths/weaknesses of the products or their success or failures

Action points on making searches are coming up later; first some information on each of these resource groups.

Security/technology review websites

Every year, different security review websites offer their opinions on what is the best computer security software. This is one of the easiest and fastest ways to find information on the latest and best options.

An example of an internet search you can make to find the latest of these articles is as follows:

"best security software for computers in 20XX"

> In place of XX add the correct year
> Optionally add the OS of your computer
> Use "antivirus" instead of "security software" per your preference

---

Terminology refresh – operating system

The operating system (OS), is the overarching software on your computer, phone or tablet that connects the hardware of these devices to all other programs you have installed so that they can run. Examples include Windows, macOS, Chrome OS and Linux. Some security products are built for multiple OSs, and some more exclusively to one or other OS. Either way, adding the OS to your search can help you filter your options.

Websites of the products

After narrowing down options, look for the direct website of the products you want to look further at. Check for the following:

• More details on how the software works
• Demos
• Pricing and different purchase options (examples: number of licenses, add-on products)
• Free trial options

Articles on the strengths/weaknesses of the products

You can compare this stage to when you are narrowing down the options in purchasing the best new television or washing machine. You first get an idea of what you want, then you narrow down to the specifics you would like to see, then filter further until you find a product that will last, is reliable and will be value for money. With security software it is just that your primary search parameter should be finding a best-in-class product to protect your practice from cyberattacks.

• Look for user reviews or issues discussed online by searching for a product you have narrowed down by name plus "vulnerabilities" or "issues" or "reviews". Evaluate if the results impact your decision-making
• Bear in mind that no product is perfect. All of them have gaps and vulnerabilities that can be found by cybercriminals; the point is, how does the product rate overall, how fast is the brand/software company at reacting to new risks and how actively does it communicate this and its latest product features too

• AV Test (https://www.av-test.org/en/antivirus/), an independent research institute in Germany, at the time of writing offers monthly updated reviews on what it evaluates as the best anti-virus for Android, macOS and Windows – for business and home set-ups. These are under the "tests" section of the institute's website. The scoring is in a simple format that is easy to follow. Subscribing to the newsletter is one way to have a reminder of when new information has been posted (AV Test, 2022). Bear in mind that the institute has not evaluated all products in the market, but resources like this might add some information towards your decision making

---

Filtering results

Always look for the latest articles when you do the internet searches mentioned throughout this book. This means that, after you click search, ensure to filter the results so that you see at the top the most recently published articles.

Most browsers will allow you to select a time frame. Such as last day, week, month(s), year(s), always. To give one example, on Google Chrome, once a search is entered, click on the "Tools" button that appears; then a selection box for time should appear on the left-hand side. If you do not know how to perform this type of filtering for the browser(s) you use, simply make an internet search for "internet search results filtering" and add the name of your browser.

First filter to see results over the last 3–6 months, then extend this up to a year if you do not get many results or would like to see older history. As your clients are relying on you to keep their interactions and data private, remember the best product is the one that is best-in-class for your device(s) at the time of purchase.

How to choose?

If the information coming next is relatively new to you, as you are a beginner, do take a deep breath and be assured that none of this will be very technical or complicated. As humans we spend a lot of time protecting things in our lives – property, other people, animals, even sandcastles that we build on the beach. You are also capable of protecting your use of the cyberspace. As you read through this book, more will become clear and the different puzzle pieces will fit together.

Narrowing down product choice

Check the reviews and articles you find to note who exactly is behind them. Make sure that it is a reputable source. Many of the articles you find might also have affiliate links to products. That said, at the end of the day, one advantage of reviews is that they do create a good summary of the pros and cons of a software, so it is easier for comparisons across them.

As a practitioner working with confidential client data, the following are some of the things to look for when choosing security software:

- **Real-time protection** – your main security software should run in real time. You can download extra products to do extra scans periodically and remove threats after they are on the PC, but you need one real-time product running at all times
- **Top of the range product** – your product should be one that is listed consistently as best-in-class. It should be a software company you can see is constantly updating against any new threats, and that the software is actively competitive against similar products. This indicates a company wanting to keep up with threats in the cyberspace and being the best at what it does
- **Clear dashboard or user functionality** – choose a product you find easy to use. By using a product for a trial period, you will quickly be able to find out if the dashboard, reports and functions are set out in a way that you can understand and use. You should be able to read the reports, know how to schedule scans and be able to run deeper/extra scans when you need to
- **Firewall** – this protects your internet connections, both in- and outbound
- **Malware protection** – one of the main cyberthreats that practitioners should be aware about is malware, which will be covered in more detail in Chapter 5. Ransomware, discussed in some of the case studies so far, is a form of malware. You should look for a product that provides excellent protection from this – on a real-time basis. Malware can enable cybercriminals to gain access to your computer, access your files and, potentially, also your banking information
- **Extras** – some products include different extras that might be considered when choosing a tool. Take care not to let the extras and advertising sway the decision, always ensure the main, core product you are purchasing is the one that will protect you best in the first instance. Extras can always be purchased later and even as standalone products from other companies if you find one with a better version. Examples include the following:
  - VPN – VPN will not be recommended in this book as it is tricky. VPN can help protect your privacy online, but it's impact against cyberattacks is usually limited and a trustworthy VPN service is usually expensive (Migliano, 2021). If you feel tempted by the advertisements around VPN, take care to inform yourself on both views and take great care with free and low-quality VPNs as many are not safe and may increase your risk of exposure to malware and viruses (Vasconcellos, 2021)
  - Cloud storage – it is not a threat detection tool, but a way to back up and store documents. You may already have it through other products you use, so check this first

- Browser guards – these are extremely valuable tools to consider. Many practitioners are very active with CPD online, attending webinars, training and downloading new information. Some are also researchers. Browser guards vary in functionality (per the product you choose) but all aim to protect your use of the internet. Often, they have options such as a small pop-up confirmation that a download appears safe, or they block websites that appear insecure
- Other extras offered by a security software provider – check what they are and if of relevance to you

Another tip for your research is that it is possible to find a lot of good reports and comparisons already made by others by typing into an internet search "comparison of x product and y product". In place of x and y, add the products you have narrowed down to and want to compare, and see what comes back. This type of search can be used to compare paid and free versions of a product as well.

Combining tools

It can be tricky to have two or more main security software products on a computer as they sometimes try to cancel each other out or block each other. One reason for this is where the products see each other as competitors (Rasch, 2019). Another reason is that they are trying to ensure you have not installed two products performing the exact same functions that need to operate in the same part of your system, as this can cause either or both of them to fail. So, if you are tempted to apply more than one main security product always research first whether the products can function together.

Alternatively, however, there are today a growing number of products that can be downloaded that can complement the main product used. Let's call these "add-on" tools. Some add-on tools that people often consider a free or paid version of are as follows:

Adware removal tool
Spyware scanner
Browser guard
Extra malware protection
Cleaners

The last – device cleaner – is not a typical security tool but can help keep a computer clean of residual items or files that might enable a threat. Cleaners can help remove among other things browser cookies, leftover files from deleted or removed items and outdated software. Often, this also enables the computer to work faster afterwards. There are some robust free products in this area. To research them, make a similar search as before, just replacing anti-virus/security software with device cleaners.

Free software

Many anti-virus and security products are offered for free or have a reduced free version. In considering any of these, carefully review what the "free" part means. Check what is missing compared with the full service and which features/options are not included. Also read the terms and conditions carefully – are they gathering and selling your data to generate income and if so – which data?

Often, free versions don't operate in real time, and the computer scan may have to be run manually. As a practitioner promising confidentiality to your clients, the bottom line is that you need an effective, best-in-class core security software product running on all your devices at all times – so scanning in real time. Free products might still, however, add value, where they are used as an extra, add-on tool to perform particular scans. Be careful when downloading any free product – only do so after having verified it thoroughly and make sure that you have checked where you are downloading the product from, as sometimes they are put up on open platforms which may not be secure.

User scenario case studies: selecting and combining tools

None of the user case studies in this section are being provided as blueprints in any way, some in fact should elicit some critique from you, particularly if you have some knowledge of cybersecurity already or are reading this book for a second time after gaining some experience. Use these as idea/reflection generators and to get insight into how unique choosing products might be. Evaluate if you feel their coverage sounds sufficient for someone working with confidential data and what you might do differently if you were the user mentioned.

User A runs a security software product popular for Mac users. They have a full licence, and they do not use any other products. However, the user has been looking at extra tools against spyware, now that their children have iPhones, and looking at products that they can leverage the licence across their Macs and all their iPhones to keep work and home data safer.

User B runs Windows Defender (free), selected on the basis of its good test score from an independent IT research institute (AV Test, 2022). User B also has a licence for another tool, which provides extra real-time malware scanning and a browser guard. In addition, they have a computer cleaning tool set-up that periodically removes unused files and software. They pay for the extra tools annually. As they work with a lot of very senior, high-profile CEOs, some under NDAs, they frequently review the software they use. User B has considered using a system that will enable clients to book directly and to also store client information and session notes going forward, but has not yet found a product they feel is secure enough, given the clients they work with. For now, User B's assistant manages bookings and runs a complex anonymisation system for all client data (more on topics like this in Chapter 8).

User C received a number of calls from Microsoft, saying that the company wants to help them fix his computer. They were aware from seeing this on television that it was a scam. Worried about any other threat "getting in", User C bought a comprehensive full-spectrum security product that also fully scans anything they do on the internet and screens all emails. The licence allows them to use the same product on all their devices and has a clear user dashboard. They also set up a free computer cleaner, which they run each weekend.

User D has a new computer and just realised they haven't thought about security software. They look up the security centre of their PC and can see it is running a product that was on the PC, on free trial. They decide to check online and find out that the product is well-rated, but they can see another product that delivers two more security features for around the same price and provides more licences for other devices in the same household. They mark on their calendar to switch to this product when the free trial finishes.

User E has completed the annual review of their security software and has seen a product rated about the same as the one they have but whose dashboard looks really easy to use. They have not actively used their current product as it feels a bit clunky and the functions do not make a lot of sense. The alternative product has three different versions, and User E decides to try one of the more advanced ones as the company has a year-end sale on, so User E can get it at the same price as their current product. User E's client list has expanded, and they think it would be great to feel that all client data is better secured than it is today. User E signs up for a trial first, to be sure that they don't get stuck again with something they don't actively use.

User F, after reading everything so far in this book and doing some research, still feels unsure about which product to choose. They consider hiring a professional to help but then recall that their nephew is always glued to computer games. Upon asking, it turns out that User F's nephew is excited to do some research on how to protect a PC and tablet. User F's nephew has some cybersecurity knowledge from college and understands the importance of his relative protecting their confidential client data. He finds and demonstrates how to install and use a product that is both best-in-class and easy to use. User F quickly picks up everything under their nephew's guidance, helped by his reassurance that if User F worked out how to use a tablet, then this will not be more difficult!

User G works as a researcher alongside being a practitioner. They use their own laptop computer. User G recently had problems with their internet browser – they had clicked on a link that had introduced a virus that changed the home page to something unpleasant. User G decided to stick with the free software on their Window's computer, but has now also installed a couple of extra tools, including a browser guard and a free adware scanner that User G has a reminder on their calendar to run every couple of days. User G has also booked an appointment to talk to IT at the company they research for to get their advice for going forward.

Pause for reflection

Make some notes on your user scenario today, and what that might need to evolve to, before moving to the checklist and action points in the next section.

Checklist: PC security software

It is time now to put down the book and go do the research indicated. As you research, get used to any new language, so that each time you review your products, you can go a little deeper and be a little more secured.

Beginners: it is recommended that you research and pick up a robust, full-service product that can cover you well. Over time, you can build up from there.

Intermediate–Advanced: use this time to start to become acquainted with potential add-on tools, such as the aforementioned or others you find.

Action 1:

- Run an internet search to review the security software options for your PC (use the search examples provided earlier)

Action 2:

- Review what you find against what you use today. Investigating alternatives builds your knowledge base. Is there anything that may provide more security for your practice?

Action 3:

- Decide on the product you want to use going forward and install it (if there is a change). Install a trial version if there is one until you are sure this is the right product for you
- If you decide to change products but want to wait until the licence of your current one expires, put this firmly on your calendar and check whether there are any extra add-on tools available that can fill the gap until then

Action 4:

- Explore the product you are using (whether you continued with an existing one or changed it). Ensure you know how the dashboard and functionality works. Check on the product website or more generally online for demos, as needed. Adjust the settings and make the most of its features. Make sure it is set to perform regular full scans as well as ongoing monitoring

Action 5:

- Create a calendar entry to review all your security products annually. Set it for 30 days prior to any licences expiring, giving you time to review and cancel an existing product if you decide to take a new one. Add in the calendar entry the steps you will undertake and the page numbers to refer to in this book, so that all you will have to do is open the reminder and go through the points. It goes without saying that you can re-assess your products more frequently than annually; however, this is a basic starting point

Action 6:

• Research add-on (p. 33) tools that might further protect your practice

Ongoing behaviours

Let's summarise the rationale and outcome of the previous pages and round up with showing that much of this has been about behaviour change as well as choosing security products. Even if this book recommended, by name, a number of security software products, those products may not stay as the top ones to use. This is why performing annual reviews is on the checklist that you just completed, implementing a new behaviour of taking responsibility for your device security on an ongoing basis.

This is important as your security will only be as good as the effort you put into it. Each time you review your security products, helps to achieve the following:

• Keeps you up to date with the market trends as well as provides information towards making the best possible choice for your practice
• Enables you to discover if another product has developed new prevention and mitigation capabilities, whereas yours has not
• Provides a chance to see if another product is more affordable and covers the same (or better) overall on the threat spectrum, enabling evaluation on whether you are getting the best value for money
• Offers a chance to try other products – perhaps one that is more intuitive to use, has an easier-to-use dashboard or works better for your needs

Remember that these products also cover your personal use of the device(s) they are on. Overall, then, you should now be sold – that a few small research tasks every twelve months will be worth the effort!

Final tips

If you find security software expensive or are not sure you want to pay a little extra for a more advanced product, note that security software, just like anything else out there, has sales offers. Look up the company's website around sales seasons and there are often some great offers. This can also be worth trying for add-on tools as well. For example, someone keen to supplement their security – with an extra tool more specifically targeting malware, adware detection or providing a computer cleaner, spyware or browser guard – might also find a good offer on a product they are interested to try out. It goes without saying, however, that a computer must at all times be protected with security software, so do not wait for a sale to get coverage in place!

Most products do have trial periods, so if you are uncertain about them, try them out before you buy. A product you find clunky or difficult to use will be one you may struggle to get optimum use from and thus fail to respond to any alerts or results in scans. When choosing and trialling a product, check that you get a sense of comfort from the way it looks, feels and operates, including that it has a dashboard you feel able to use to set scans of your computer that return reports you can read.

Please don't be alarmed when you get reports or notifications from your tools either. Remember it's your software doing its job. Stay calm and read through what it is and take steps from there. If it is a minor threat, your security suite will have options to quarantine and solve it; if it is a major threat, you may need to consider the actions that come later in Chapter 5.

Note that each product you implement (main security software or add-ons) will return alerts differently, so you will need to learn separately how each works. This will come with time and use.

Author's experience

When my browser guard says it has blocked a website I have tried to open, my first reaction is often a nervous one: what exactly have I clicked on! Then I regroup – it is my software doing its job (blocking the site). I pause to have a second think about why I clicked on that link and if I have been careful in my choice to do so. I also remember that sometimes the blocking is due to the website simply having poor security rather than there being something malicious waiting for me there. Whatever the reason, the block is for my own good, and when this happens, I move on to other websites and do not pursue ways around the blocking.

Having a product that can alert me about the websites I click on has had a second benefit. It reminds me to be careful. It's easy to get complacent that everything is fine, that my computer is covered and thus fall for an exciting title or bit of information that I have been looking for and click a little too quickly.

Mark's case – Part 2

In Part 1, we got to know Mark. To take a break before moving on to talk about other devices than PCs, let's have another look at his case. If you need to, quickly re-read through what happened to Mark in Part 1 (p. 14).

Mark prides himself on being rather diligent when it comes to cybersecurity. He is aware that clicking on a link can lead to all kinds of problems. He also knows that a get-rich-scheme is probably a scam. The problem is that on the right day, the "right" story can slide into your life and make sense to you in a way that red flags just don't come into view. Everyone is at risk of falling for the story being unfolded for them by a criminal or fraudster when that happens. This is where human factors come in, and you will train your responses and reactions through reading the case studies in this book and undertaking the reflective activities.

Here is some extra information towards evaluating what has happened in Mark's case:

Timing

If tax had called Mark another time of year, he would have answered the phone a little confused and wondering what was up. They were calling at a time of year businesses were active with tax returns.

Spoofing

Mark received a call that showed up on his phone as "tax authorities". Let's briefly cover the different types of spoofing fraudsters use:

Phone number spoofing (caller ID spoofing)

A number dialling you is masked by another number, meaning that the number on your screen appears to be one from your area or from an authority or a service provider that you know.

SMS spoofing

A message appears to come from a number you know, perhaps has the name of a company on it, but the original sender is masked.

Spoofed emails

The sender of the email uses a spoofed email address which looks similar to the email address of a company you hear from frequently. There are often small differences to the original, such as changes in the case of a letter (upper/lower), missing or added characters, for example, notifications@onedrive1.com, info@PayPAL.com, or subtle changes to the writing script, for example, PayPal.com, googIe.com or *G00GLE.COM* (examples cited by IDN homograph attack, 2021). Along with this, often the display name may still show perfectly as the company name, for example: "PayPal".

Spoofed websites

You guessed it: these are websites that look like the original versions. As with anything, quality – when it comes to spoofing – can vary. Some spoofing will be easy to spot, while others will be very hard to detect because of very subtle differences to the original that anyone can easily overlook. Again, subtle changes – such as changes in use of lower or uppercase letters, a slight difference in format, colour, name – may give something away. With spoofing that is done well a login screen can also look as it always does and ask for the same information. This is why it is important to always have an instinct for when something is not quite right.

Use your instincts.

If you note something does not feel right, do not push that feeling away.

Meaning: listen to yourself. Don't be afraid to pause, look a little deeper, read a little more carefully, listen more closely. Always take the time to double-check/ research if what you are responding to is legitimate. We will unpack this more in Chapters 3, 6 and 7.

Activity

Take out your reflective notes. With everything you have now read in Mark's case – Part 1 and 2, what red flags do you now think are present in the story? We will continue with the final part in Chapter 3.

Mobile device security software (phones and tablets)

So far, we have covered the need to protect our computers and the importance of our choices in how we do that. The same needs, however, apply to all the other electronic devices that we use online. We will focus on smartphones and tablets in this section.

Security software

Anti-virus and security software for your mobile devices is typically downloaded as a "mobile security", "mobile anti-virus" or "mobile security and anti-virus" app. To research and decide on the one that is best for your mobile devices, you will need to know the OS of the device. You might have an affinity towards a particular brand and your PC, mobile and tablet might all be from this brand and they may be using the same OS. Or, you may choose your devices on the basis of what you think is the best brand for that device or is a good price at that time. It is therefore entirely possible that some readers have a tablet that may be iOS, a phone that may be Android and a PC that is something entirely different, like Chrome OS. You can only download and use a mobile security product that is built for the OS of your mobile device.

If you don't know what the OS is for your mobile devices, you can look up the hardware on the device itself or you can check your manual or the manufacturer's website.

To decide the optimum security products for mobile devices, use the same resources as for computers:

1. security/technology review websites
2. websites of the products
3. articles on the strengths/weaknesses of the products or their success or failures

The purpose of each of the three groups is the same as for the computer section, so review those pages as needed. The following is an example of the internet search you can make to find the latest of these articles:

"best antivirus for mobile devices in 20XX" or "best security software for mobile devices in 20XX"

> in place of XX, add the correct year

Either add your OS (android, iOS, other) into your search or filter through the results for your OS.

The checklist coming up in a couple of pages will guide you through the actions to take.

How to choose?

When you make your decisions on which product to use, check if the security suite you have for your PC covers other devices, and if it does, review if it will be adequate also for your phone/tablet.

Other factors in deciding which product:

• Consider how much you work on the mobile device. If you work a lot directly from your tablet or phone, particularly on client-related information, you

need to take this into consideration when choosing security products that will protect your data adequately
- If you make a lot of calls, use cloud storage accessed from the device, write emails or texts to clients from it, then this should also inform your choices

Don't be tempted to skip protecting mobile devices. The way we use mobile devices can be very click and go, as they are products designed to make our lives easier. So, we may click more, check less and see fewer red flags on a mobile device compared to when we sit at a computer. At the same time, we are using these devices more and more for "sensitive and critical tasks" (Bubukayr & Almaiah, 2021), so do take your time going through this review and finding the right security product(s) for your mobile devices. In the next chapter, we will also look at networks and how any device on a network essentially can bring vulnerabilities to everything else on the same network. Your network will be as weak as its weakest link – don't make that link a mobile or tablet with no (or inadequate) security!

Checklist mobile/tablet security software

Put this into action before moving on to the next part of the chapter.

Action 1:

- Run an internet search to review the best security software for your mobile and, if applicable, tablet. Ensure to check for the relevant OS of each device.

Action 2:

- Review what you find against what you use today.

Action 3:

- Decide on the product you want to use going forward and install it (if there is a change). Install a trial version if there is one until you are sure this is the right product for you.
- If you decide to change products but want to wait until the licence of your current one expires, put this firmly on your calendar and check whether there are any extra add-on tools available that can fill the gap until then.

Action 4:

- Explore the product you are using (whether you continued with an existing one or changed it). Ensure you know how the dashboard and functionality works, adjust the settings and features.

Action 5:

- Ensure you add to the calendar entry you already created to review your PC security software to do the same for your mobile devices.

Security tips – all devices

In Chapter 3, coming up next, we look at networks, passwords and topics around the use of a device. The rest of this chapter continues to focus on securing the device itself and explores ways to do this beyond security software.

Password/biometrics on the device

Many tablets and OS now have the user set up an account to open and operate the PC or device. Where possible, make use of any biometrics options for signing into this account: fingerprint, voice recognition or face recognition. Biometrics can be breached – anything can – for example, criminals are exchanging fingerprint emulation tools on the darknet (Paganini, 2021), but biometrics are still currently more secure than a single log-on password. Having no lock on your device means that it is an easy target for anyone in the vicinity of your device and can gain them unauthorised access to your client data. It is vital therefore that – when you are not using your device – it is locked, even if you have stepped away from it just briefly.

Stolen device

Many devices have options to track them if they are stolen or missing – and you can set that up either using the tracking software the device suggests or using another app. Before you set up any such, research again, because you do need to be sure you are opting to enable a reputable tracker. This is important for it will be essentially tracking your device and storing that information. Review exactly what it will have access to and what information it will store, too. Bear in mind that a seasoned thief is aware of how to disable any tracking software.

We will also discuss cloud storage in Chapter 8, but worth adding here is one advantage of using cloud storage: some offer a "remote wipe" service that may enable that all the files on a stolen device are deleted the next time it is online. PC tracking software may offer similar capabilities. Depending on how the criminal who has your device operates, they may seek out the data available on the PC before they go online, and you may not have a chance for this to work, but it will always be worth a try. If you have cloud storage, check the product pages to see if they offer this service in your subscription. Familiarise yourself with how it works, so that you have some basic idea of what to do if there was a need to. If you want to check more generally which cloud services offer remote wipe, then just do an internet search on "cloud storage providers with remote wipe". Some mobile devices themselves may also have a remote wipe option, where the whole device can be wiped if required. As mentioned before, ensure to research what is offered thoroughly before installing.

If a device issued to you by a corporate or an educational institution (or any other third party) is stolen, you should of course ring the relevant IT or security team there for advice on the next steps. If your device is your own, but linked to the network of a corporation or an educational institution (or any other third party), you should still contact them as they may be able to help or prevent data loss. Similarly, if you experience any cyberattack on a device provided by a third party or a device linked to a third-party network, you will need to inform them without delay.

Downloading apps

When downloading apps on any device always take care only to download from a trusted store or site. If you are downloading something very new to you that you have also not really heard of before, cross-check it online. How many have downloaded an app is usually displayed alongside reviews. There is also a checklist at the end of this book to remind of some basic steps around apps.

Importance of updates on any device

It is not always optimal timing when your computer flashes a message that it wants to run updates, especially if you have just started something or have a lot of documents and programs open. However, it is important to take on a view that all the programs, software, systems you use are not static – they evolve; therefore, they do need updating.

Mobile devices tend to be easier to update, the updates often run faster, and apps are easier to open again afterwards.

Updates you will likely experience on the devices that you use as a practitioner relate to the following:

- Firmware
- OS
- Video conferencing software
- Security products
- Other software (might include Microsoft Office, apps, browsers, CRMs, booking systems and other programs used to provide services)
- Drivers

Updates enable the following

- Patching security weaknesses
- Enhancing or adding to a product's security
- Improving efficiency and optimisation
- Installing new features
- Updating features

Many updates are created to mitigate threats that cybercriminals are exploiting. Delaying updating your computer or device will leave it vulnerable. In addition to the security side of updates, they are often about performance as well, and may introduce improved or new services. Reframe the friction of restarting a device by considering it as a virtual coffee break for your technology and taking a break yourself as everything installs.

Note that many internet browsers update automatically, but changes may not all apply until they are restarted. So don't be tempted to leave browsers open for days on end; it will leave you vulnerable (Kingsley-Hughes, 2021).

Older operating systems

Earlier, we looked at how the pride some people have in not being online can backfire, where someone may take over your digital imprint for you (Krebs, 2020). Similarly, every so often there is an OS that people don't take to, and they try to hang onto the one before as long as possible.

Perhaps some of you reading this were not fans of Windows Vista, for example. The problem is that OSs are situated in the cybersecurity arms race. When OSs get old, they are not updated as frequently as the newer versions are. As a result, they often become targets for criminals. Holding on to very outdated software can increase the risk of cyber incidents and data breaches on your computer (NCSC, 2020, 2021). Hanging on to an old OS as a practitioner handling confidential data might not be something to be proud of. The same goes for old internet browsers and any older product. Whether you want to hear it or not, the truth is that it is only by participating and staying on track in the cyber arms race that you can keep your practice as safe as possible.

New OSs are also not impervious. Although they go through extensive testing, it is usually impossible to detect and remove all defects (Alhazmi et al., 2007). Criminals look for vulnerabilities and defects in new OSs as well as older ones, but the difference is that newer/updated versions will normally still be safer and have more attention from its developers if something does arise.

If you have a very old or older OS on your computer, you may want to check how vulnerable it is now from attack and how frequently it still gets security fixes. To check vulnerability, perform a simple internet search as follows:

X <name of OS> + vulnerabilities

> add the name of the OS of your computer in place of X
> remember as always to filter your results to see the latest first

The results should show you the latest vulnerabilities for your OS.

If you, for any reason, continue to use a very old OS, browser or any software that has a number of current vulnerabilities and/or could be considered obsolete due to it no longer being supported by its manufacturer, be aware that your decision to use it will put your client data at extra risk. As a minimum, do some research on how you can take some steps that can help reduce that (NCSC, 2019, 2021).

Reframing

The next time you need to run updates to a product, or buy a new version, reframe the view. Try not to see it as friction, effort and money spend. See it instead as a necessary part of your business practice. Just as you need to work on your accounts, keep records of your clients, implement legislation related to business practices, you also need to invest money and time into the tools you use.

Look at obtaining new software as an all-round investment. As software changes, it grows in complexity, so new versions are learning experiences and the sooner we get used to new features, the better, as typically the day when we have to will come anyway. It may also perform better and be easier to use. Just as you change parts in a car to keep it running optimally, so that it can keep you safe on the road, you also need to change "parts" related to your devices to keep you and your clients safe from cyber harm.

For those of you who like data, Microsoft releases security updates every month. In January 2022 alone, Microsoft patched 120 security holes across its software products and windows systems (Krebs, 2022). Updates strengthen your fortress walls, correcting errors or fixing holes that cybercriminals have found (or will find) and are exploiting to gain access to people's worlds.

Most OSs publish their updates; just search for the "OS + security updates" to find their webpage. These can be difficult to read but give a picture of how regularly a product is being updated. Examples:

Apple: https://support.apple.com/en-us/HT201222

Microsoft: https://msrc.microsoft.com/update-guide

Summary

Among other topics, this chapter covered the following:

*   Informed of the importance of researching security software that protects your devices
*   Taught how to research this on a regular basis, so that your devices are always covered with the best-possible security software
*   Clarified the importance of considering all devices – PC, tablet and phone
*   Provided a reminder on the importance of protecting entry/access to the devices

---

Activity

Revisit the answers you wrote in your reflective notes to the questions at the start of the chapter. Add to your notes how you would answer the questions now. The next chapter will look at the networks we use our devices over and also security around logging into anything we have access credentials for.

References

Alhazmi, O. H., Malaiya, Y. K., & Ray, I. (2007). Measuring, analyzing and predicting security vulnerabilities in software systems. *Computers & Security*, *26*(3), 219–228. https://doi.org/10.1016/j.cose.2006.10.002

Apple. (n.d.). *Apple security updates.* https://support.apple.com/en-us/HT201222

AV Test. (2022). *Tests.* https://www.av-test.org/en/antivirus/

Bubukayr, M. A. S., & Almaiah, M. A. (2021). Cybersecurity concerns in smart-phones and applications: A survey. *2021 International Conference on Information Technology (ICIT)*, 725–731. https://doi.org/10.1109/ICIT52682.2021.9491691.

IDN Homograph Attack. (2021, May 3). *In Wikipedia.* https://en.wikipedia.org/wiki/IDN_homograph_attack

Kingsley-Hughes, A. (2021, June 14). *Here's why you should restart Google Chrome at least once a week.* ZDnet. https://www.zdnet.com/article/heres-why-you-should-restart-google-chrome-at-least-once-a-week/

Krebs, B. (2020, August 12). *Why and where you should plant your flag.* Krebs on Security. https://krebsonsecurity.com/2020/08/why-where-you-should-you-plant-your-flag/

Krebs, B. (2022, January 11). *'Wormable' Flaw Leads January 2022 Patch Tuesday.* Krebs on Security. https://krebsonsecurity.com/2022/01/wormable-flaw-leads-january-2022-patch-tuesday/

Microsoft. (n.d.). *Security update guide.* https://msrc.microsoft.com/update-guide

Migliano, S. (2021, December 30). *The 10 disadvantages of using a VPN.* Top10VPN. https://www.top10vpn.com/what-is-a-vpn/vpn-disadvantages/

National Cyber Security Centre. (2019, January 19). *End user device (EUD) security guidance.* Crown Copyright. https://www.ncsc.gov.uk/collection/end-user-device-security/securing-obsolete-platforms

National Cyber Security Centre. (2020, January 17). *Weekly threat report 17th January 2020.* Crown Copyright. https://www.ncsc.gov.uk/report/weekly-threat-report-17th-january-2020

National Cyber Security Centre. (2021, June 21). *Device security guidance.* Crown Copyright. https://www.ncsc.gov.uk/collection/mobile-device-guidance/managing-the-risks-from-obsolete-products

Paganini, P. (2021, June 15). *Wear your MASQ! New device fingerprint spoofing tool available in dark web.* Security Affairs. https://securityaffairs.co/wordpress/118981/cyber-crime/masq-fingerprint-spoofing-tool.html

Rasch, M. (2019, December 6). *Can antivirus companies use "Good Samaritan" defense to block rival software?* Security Boulevard. https://securityboulevard.com/2019/12/can-antivirus-companies-use-good-samaritan-defense-to-block-rival-software/

Vasconcellos, E. (2021, June 30). *What are the pros and cons of VPNs?* Business.com. https://www.business.com/vpn/pros-cons/

Chapter 3

Networks, login credentials and embracing friction

Introduction

By the end of the chapter, the reader will understand the importance of a secure network and of strong login credentials, such as MFA and biometrics, in a world where passwords are no longer enough. This forms another layer in our cybersecurity defences. In this chapter, we also touch on how using our homes to work can cause vulnerabilities and make our cybersecurity less secure. Even if you work in a separate space in your home, your environment may be full of distractions (chores, other people) that can make you unfocused and less attentive to red flags. This can make you an easier target for cybercriminals and fraudsters (Okereafor & Manny, 2020). The chapter also covers tips on how to share home network access with visitors/guests, and a deep-dive into the risks around buying and using second-hand devices.

Topics that will be covered include the following:

Networks
Routers
Public Wi-Fi
Passwords
MFA
Second-hand and older devices

The chapter will build the following:

Awareness

Of the very basics of security regarding

Networks
Routers
Public Wi-Fi

DOI: 10.4324/9781003184805-4

Understanding

Of important information pertaining to

Login credentials
Securing all devices on a network
Second-hand and older devices

Improved practices

Related to

Protecting your client data, including more secure practices around the use of networks and login credentials

A written book cannot fully replace hands-on help, so when in any doubt about anything in this chapter or book, do consult a professional.

*

Routers and networks

First, a little terminology. Networks essentially connect devices together, enabling devices to send and receive data between each other. Most home networks connect to and use the internet to do this transmission. The terms "internet" and "Wi-Fi" are often used synonymously by people, perhaps because due to the prevalence of Wi-Fi today. They are, however, not the same thing – the internet being the overarching global network through which information can be sent from one network (or device) to another and Wi-Fi being the technology that essentially enables your devices to connect wirelessly, via radio waves, to each other (Norton, 2022). Routers are the hardware that route data and traffic, from the devices in your home to the wider internet.

Basics on securing routers

When you install an internet router (to connect to the internet), it has a password. This is not your internet login password but the password that is on your router account. Always ensure your router has a unique, strong password that it is not the default username/password that it came with.

To reset a router and its password, log into the router online using the current details if you have them. Alternatively, many routers have a reset button on them and from there you can revert to the instructions for your router to restart to factory settings. Search online how to reset the router you have (add name and model to your search) if you do not have the original instructions. If you are more technical, one way to log in is via the default gateway IP. This can be found via command prompt (Hoffman, 2017), or many routers have the IP 192.168.1.1 or 192.168.2.1. If you paste either of those sets of numbers into a web browser and receive a login screen, then you have one of those. This website, https://cirt.net/passwords – has also logged the IPs and router default passwords for most manufacturers (CIRT,

2021). If you find you can log in using the default password for your router, reset your router immediately applying a new, unique, strong password as well as take that as a stark reminder to never keep the default password any device comes with ever again!

Top reminders:

- Always create a complex router password
- Use a unique password – do not use a password you use on anything else

Do not use old routers

Older routers may no longer be security patched by their manufacturers (Wakefield, 2021). Not only will a newer router be safer, it will also operate faster and more efficiently. So, while it can feel like an outlay to replace it every few years, it will be worth it. As with security software, to find a good, secure router, you can search online to find the latest reviews (example search: "most secure internet router 20XX") which often help pinpoint new router features and extra controls you might find interesting (Delaney, 2021).

Your home network

While it is tempting to set up your internet network name to something that matches your business name, or the name of your house, flat number, surname or any other that makes it clear it is "yours", this can also draw attention to your network. "Janet_Taylor_Counselling" will sound like a more interesting target for hackers than a group of random letters and numbers. Once on your network, someone with the experience will look for ways into the devices on it.

Important:

- Create a complex Wi-Fi password
- Do not make your password a copy of your network name or something simple that anyone with information about you can guess
- Do not use a password you use on anything else
- Update the password periodically
- If you are more advanced or ready to go deeper, check whether the router, OS or any other software you have offers more security tools around your use of the internet. For example, some routers have settings to help prevent remote access

Public Wi-Fi

You can become a victim of a cyberattack or cyber-enabled fraud outside of your practice network – on any network you connect to. Public Wi-Fi is high risk for both your personal and business data. Very simply, do not ever, as a practitioner, use public Wi-Fi. This includes a warning never to use public Wi-Fi with a device you do not use with clients/has no link to your client data, but that you later will re-connect to a network with devices you do use with clients.

As a practitioner, always consider having your own solution for accessing the internet when outside of the workplace or home office, that is, always aim to avoid using an external network of any kind.

When using a laptop/tablet outside of the workplace and provided your mobile phone is securely covered by an anti-virus and is up-to-date – you can hotspot internet from your mobile phone plan to your computer/tablet. When you open a hotspot via your phone, always enable a password on it – never open a hotspot without a complex, strong password, as anyone looking up networks in the region you are in will otherwise be able to use it.

Despite giving this solution on using a hotspot, it goes without saying to take care with this. While it may sound very adventurous, for example, to work on your laptop at a cafe, do remember the following:

1. Always still take care not to type up client notes or other confidential materials where others can read them on your screen
2. Using a phone hotspot is not quite as secure as using your own network – the security on your phone is very likely not as good as that of a device connected directly to a secure home router. So, if you do not need to connect your laptop/device to the internet, don't

For tablets, check if your mobile network provider can supply extra SIM cards as an add-on to your current plan. Sometimes, this option is not so expensive.

For those still tempted by public Wi-Fi, perhaps some more information may help dissuade you. First, note that an open access network, where you do not need to use a password, is particularly insecure – you will be on the same network as everyone else linked to the same open access. Hackers prey on such set-ups, which enable them to intercept data sent to and from the devices people have connected to them. Don't also be tempted by public Wi-Fi where the user needs to set up an account and a password. This is still an unknown network with often unclarified security and often comes with you signing off some lengthy terms and conditions to use such a service.

If you still decide to access public Wi-Fi despite the advice here, a few things to consider:

•   Read any terms and conditions. Absorb what precisely happens to the data on your device when you sign up and accept the terms
•   Ensure you are clear on the implications for you if something happens – revisit any legislation you are obliged to follow for your location and profession

- Consider how you can mitigate the risk. This might include scanning your laptop and removing the network connection fully from the device after use
- Never create a public WiFi account – using a password you use on anything else. Consider also setting up a second email you use to register for such services, rather than using your business/usual one (form yourself an alias)

To be clear: these points above will not protect you against a well-seasoned criminal if you go ahead and use an insecure network.

Our roles as counsellors, therapists and coaches include safeguarding client data and privacy. This means never putting these at risk. While we can all appreciate something that comes for free, free internet is simply an offer that practitioners should pass on. See any extra cost as necessary operating expenses.

Using friends and family Wi-Fi

If you go to stay with people you know well for a period of time and decide to connect to their internet, with a device you use in your practice, establishing that a network is as secure as possible before connecting to it is important. It is a little awkward to ask your family and friends if they have secure internet, they might not even know. There are a few small things you can look for. A starter clue is whether the network is private and requires a password. Are the network name and password easy to figure out? This indicates that the people setting it up are not aware this makes it easier to breach – which might be a clue that the rest of the security may also not be minimal. When you connect, do not set your device to be visible by others on the network. If in any doubt about the network, use your own mobile hotspot.

Learn to love complexity!

There are few things more fiddly and irritating than imputing a strange, long, irregular password to get connected to the internet; however, each time you find yourself thinking this, reframe that it is keeping the network and anything on your devices more secure.

One-time/temporary visitors

The network you use in your office space/home to link devices that contain client information and confidential data is a network you should not give one-time or temporary visitors access to. This includes, for example, clients, someone you have hired to come perform some work or someone supplying any kind of service. Today, most people will have their own mobile phone with internet access. As therapists, counsellors, coaches, it is unlikely your client should require or need internet access while on your premises in relation to services you are providing. Other visitors, performing a trade, service or representing a company, should have their own solution to retrieve records online on any device they come with (e.g. over their phone hotspot).

It can be difficult to turn down someone from using your internet, but you can find some creative ways to do so, such as saying you "Can't remember the password right now".

If you start to consider allowing a temporary visitor onto your network (still very much not recommended), evaluate first for red flags such as the following:

- Is the person very persistent about using your internet?
- Is the purpose of them needing access here and now clear, and does it make sense?
- How unknown is the person asking this?
- Is the company they work for also relatively or fully unknown to you? Remember that a genuine company with a good IT security set-up would not want their staff using clients' potentially unsafe home networks. They would have a network solution for their staff to use when they are out of the office

Final questions to yourself before you decide:

- Are your own devices on the network fully secured and not visible to others?
- Can what the visitor needs access for actually wait?

If you still do go ahead and give them access, as a minimum ensure to run a full security scan using your main security software and change your network password afterwards.

Family and friends using your Wi-Fi

When you have known guests staying in your home and they would like to use your internet, take a responsible, informed decision on the basis of: your knowledge of the visitors, the maturity of your security and the devices your guests are connecting (how secure those devices are and how they will use them). It is, again, perhaps a little awkward to ask people you know questions about the security of their devices; however, if you run a business over a home or business network, you need to think about it. Ensure also that you have set up your network in such a way that devices on it are not visible to each other (go into internet settings from a device to check).

Some routers may allow you to set up a separate "guest" network and password. This gives some separation between your network and that of your guests. However, hackers can use this as a way in to your main network, so always give it a complex password, don't advertise the password, change it regularly and check if you can deactivate the guest network when it is not in use (some routers will offer that option).

Piggybacking and sharing internet networks

As a practitioner working with confidential data, you do need your own internet. Don't share your neighbours' internet or share your internet with them.

*

Login credentials

"Password" is the term you will all be familiar with when it comes to logging into something. "Login credentials", however, more accurately describes the information known only to us that we use to gain access to hardware, software, devices, accounts and more. These are often categorised as something you:

know (password)
have (key fob/OTP device) or
are (biometric)

In the following section, first there will be an outline of some of the issues around weak password security, followed by a discussion on the need for complex, unique passwords and a brief explanation on why MFA has been introduced. Finally, the section will offer an explanation of password managers, which are currently a way of storing passwords that some security bodies/authorities recommend.

Password apocalypse?

At points in this section, it is going to feel that the time of passwords has gone and that they are on their last lap of the stadium. This is to provide the background for why newer types and layers of login credentials, such as MFA and biometrics, have evolved and are needed. Also, bear in mind that the password is currently still the first defensive wall in your login credentials tool-kit – a wall that, through a strong password, you can make as stable as possible for the walls after it.

Simple passwords

Newspapers and websites sometimes make fun of the passwords people choose for themselves, revealing how many thousands of people are using "password" or "iloveliverpool" to log into something. Passwords like this are very easy to break (NCSC, 2019b). Therefore, over time, the requirements for the password you create to access something have become more complicated, with products themselves starting to put in rules as to what your password needs to make it a little stronger. Unfortunately, there are still many ways to crack a password (see further learning section at end for guidance, if you want to know more), meaning that "P@ssword123!" is not necessarily that much more secure than "password"; it just might take a little longer to hack. Hacked common password lists, which show exposed passwords, are easily viewable online (NCSC, 2019a, 2020a).

What should practitioners do?

There is no silver bullet of a perfect password. The problem is that cyber-criminals have so many ways to get hold of a password that ultimately, they are all fallible. That said, there are a number of things practitioners can do to ensure that best practices around passwords are implemented for improving the following:

- Protecting data pertaining to their practice
- Protecting client data
- Protecting devices
- Protecting conversations and correspondence
- Protecting software requiring a username and password to log in to use

The steps that follow provide practical tips to do this – as you read, pause and get started. Applying these will help you firm up the security of the first layer of your logging into something.

Making secure passwords

Never use the same password in more than one place

While this can feel fantastically irritating, this is possibly the most important of all rules. Once your password is breached, criminals will very likely get hold of it. It doesn't take them very long to guess other websites, places, accounts you might use and then try the same password there.

Accept the friction of different companies having different complexities of passwords

Let's face it: it can also be extremely frustrating that password requirements (length, inclusion of numbers, symbols and a mixture of upper and lowercase letters) are not universal and depend on what is set as standard by the company establishing the device, software, account or other that you are creating access to. However, they will have a reason behind their choices, and it is worth reframing each time that friction comes up.

Complexity means the product manufacturer actually has thought through how to make access more secure in a positive way.

There are also, in some countries, government agencies providing minimum guidelines for what companies need to apply as password standards (National Institute of Standards and Technology, [NIST], 2017). These tend to be fairly basic, and each company can, beyond these, still establish what it thinks is appropriately secure. This means a company that has experienced a number of breaches or attempted breaches, or that has determined security requires a higher complexity of passwords, may force users towards more complex passwords.

As of the time of writing, many government agencies, including the FBI (FBI, n.d.), actually recommend using "passphrases". These are longer passwords consisting of random words. Symbols, numbers or casing can still be part of the phrase you choose, as required/desired. You can find websites that can illuminate more on how to do this; one is https://www.useapassphrase.com/. You can also perform an internet search for "strong password checker" and find a number of tools that evaluate if a password is strong or weak. However:

- Only use tools verified as trusted. Cross-check the name of the site and who is running it
- Only use them to practice forming a strong password or passphrase. Most password checking sites/tools promise they are not storing your data, but if they have been hacked, someone else may be doing exactly that. When you form your final, actual passphrase/password, do not put that into an online tool to verify its strength. Create a final one offline, trusting that you have understood how to make it complex from your practice with the tool
- Never also use such a tool where they ask for any static data from you. They should just offer you a box to add your attempt and provide you onscreen a score after; they don't need to email it to you or know your name or address

Password storage on paper

By now you should be wondering how you will remember all your unique, strong passwords. That is fully up to you to determine. The advice to not write passwords down came around as people often would stick them right on the device they logged into, or store their pin along with their credit card in the same wallet. Today, some security experts confirm it is more about being smarter "how" you write passwords down (Krebs, n.d.).

If you are creative, you can code them in a way no one else can understand them. The trick is also to never store them in a way that it is obvious what they correspond to. Finally, never ever write them down in a document file on a device (Krebs, n.d.)! Criminals will look for this if they get onto your network or device, and they will find it (Goodin, 2021). Don't make it easy for them to log into everything. In summary: if you want to write down passwords, get imaginative and ensure that they are disguised, coded and not with you on the move.

Password managers – apps/browser extension

At the time of writing, some government agencies have actually endorsed the use of password managers (NCSC, 2018a). These are tools to store all your passwords under one master login, which can also be a fingerprint. A password manager can be on one device, for example, a single app on your phone, or it could be a service you sync across apps and browser extensions on different devices.

To find out the right one for you and your practice needs, again, this is a case of doing a little research (Laughlin, 2021). Password managers are also breached – it is important to be aware of that. So, as always, it is important to choose a high-quality, secure product. Interestingly, many security authorities point to the fact that having a password manager enables secure storage of complex, unique passwords (NCSC, 2018a). So, the risk of the password manager being breached is considered by those authorities as a lesser risk than users using easy to breach, "therapist123" type of passwords across all their accounts (FBI, n.d.).

Best practice will be to reflect on your responsibilities when using such a tool. For example, some of them allow auto-fill capabilities to relevant account login screens on your device. You will be safer if you do not use this and also if you just use a password manager on one device. If you decide to use an auto-fill feature on a password manager, you should check the settings and, as a minimum, ensure your master password is requested each time this feature is used. Where you use the password manager not only as a device app but also as a browser extension, reflect on how diligent you will be in opening and closing such a tool and protecting anything inside it from other people who are around your devices.

One tip that may be useful to those worried about the security of a password manager is to consider coding and disguising the entries. If you are good at partially remembering your passwords/phrases, one way to add them to a password manager is to include them partially or find a way to code them over different entries and not store username and password together. For example, add just enough of the password/phrase that you can remember the rest and manually add the remainder yourself. Then, you make it just that little harder for someone to use them in the event of a breach and might gain a little more time to update your passwords before someone cracks them fully (if they can).

Password managers often offer a backup service. Using this is not recommended as if you download a list of your passwords to a device, and your device is breached the information can be found by a fraudster, who will make the most of this bounty. Instead if, for any reason, you cannot access your password manager and/or the contents are lost, reset your passwords one by one as you come to use them.

Password managers – web browser

Most, if not all, web browsers offer some form of their own auto-fill password storage. However, take great care. Browsers and the passwords and data stored in them are increasingly hacked by malware (Tung, 2021). Be very aware of the vulnerabilities of having a password fully stored and ready to input in your internet browser and make an informed decision on whether it is appropriate for you to use such a tool on a device you use for your practice and with clients.

Review legislation

Ensure that use of any type of password manager does not breach any data privacy/storage/other legislation for your practice in your country of operation.

Reframing

Let's take a short pause to appreciate the friction of all of this and other parts of cybersecurity. Anyone old enough to remember only having a single stationary phone at home will know it was easy to go offline – you just took the phone off the hook! Today, going offline is just not that easy. You may be in an age bracket where the first ATM pin code you ever had might even have been 1234 or 1111. Some of the first passwords used when the internet first started were also very simple. Unfortunately, criminals quickly picked up on this. Today, for example, they will check whether you use your birth year as your pin.

Login credential complexity has come over time in response to increased criminal activity. It is why today it's typically not possible to have pin that is sequential or same digits, and password requirements have become more complex, as mentioned earlier.

The days of simple credentials are absolutely gone, and it is worth taking a moment to acknowledge the frustration. Then, let it go and accept it. Cybercriminals are not going to go backwards. With increased technology has come increased invasion from those wanting to gain from it and increased responsibility for secure use of it for the users.

This means, as a practitioner, if you want to use the latest tools and resources that enable a digitalised practice (or even in your private space), it does come with having to take on some friction to ensure security. For example, this chapter will also look at MFA, which is often perceived as extra friction. However, it is currently one of the best ways to secure your accounts.

Third-party breaches

This book helps you set up your own cybersecurity and defences. However, there will come more and more cases where you become exposed not due to your own security but that of the products, companies, brands, tools (and so forth) that you use. These are "third parties" to you. They provide something that you use to enable your practice and give good service to your customers.

Third parties with which you have accounts can be breached, and this is one way your data can also be exposed. So, for example, you use a booking system that is run by Company Z. The company experiences a cyber breach, and as a result, your client data is taken. There may be implications for you as a result. So, even with secure passwords and credentials, criminals have other ways to your data. Depending on how third-party risk develops, it may feature more in a future edition of this book. For now, know that this is the reason the book encourages a research-driven approach with ongoing reviews of the tools you decide to use. Using an insecure tool leaves you exposed, and while you cannot control how another company is storing your data or managing their operations, you can control your choice of them.

Data privacy laws in many countries now require companies to inform you if there has been a breach of your data. If you receive such an alert from a company, do ensure to read through thoroughly what is sent to you. Check what precisely was breached, and from understanding how you have been exposed, you can take steps.

Do not be alarmed by this section. The steps you learn from this book mean that you will be protecting yourself on the elements you can. For example, by not using the same password in multiple places – if a third party is breached, your password will not be re-used easily by fraudsters trying it out in other places. This will protect you to an extent from further exposure. As noted in the first chapter of this book, it can often take companies a long time to discover a breach and inform you, giving criminals time to extract your data from a third party and use it. If you have been using the same password on everything you log into and this is harvested, it may not take long for breaches to start in other places you have used it.

Action points

Often, we take a break to stretch our legs; this time, take a break to stretch your security.

Execute the following before reading further. These steps should not take very long and will start some worthwhile security behaviours. If you operate your practice on a device and/or network you also use for private use, you should consider undertaking the steps for both work and private accounts.

Passwords

1. Go to all places you are using the same password and update to a new, secure, unique password/passphrase
2. As you are updating passwords, if you are offered MFA or 2FA of any kind, enable this (this topic will be unpacked more in the next section)
3. Check any security questions you have added answers for. Don't be afraid to create an alias for yourself – with an alternative mother's maiden name, alternative street you lived on or name of a pet you wanted but didn't get. Come up with something you can remember and no one else knows or can find out about you
4. Decide if you will use a password manager to store your passwords. If yes, research the best one for you. Search for "most secure password manager, 20XX". Check out what government authorities, legislative bodies or other relevant authorities in your location have to say about password managers before you make your decision
5. When choosing a password manager, research if the product has had any breaches – just search on "product name + breach". Any of them can experience a breach; key will be how they handled it if records were exposed, and the mitigation of this going forward. If you in the future see a news article where a governmental security authority states that password managers are now unsafe, immediately re-evaluate your use of one
6. If you decide to use a password manager (or already do), make an annual calendar reminder to review if you are using the most secure product available. Set the reminder for a month before payment date if you use a paid product. When you do that annual review, check if alternative products are better options
7. Consider not to store passwords for something you very rarely log into but still need access to. Password reset functions are today usually very efficient and will typically ensure you change your password for that site at the same time as the reset. However, keep in mind that like everything else, criminals can take advantage of password resets too, so scrutinise that reset follow-up emails (links/codes) sent to you appear in order

Compromised passwords

It can be tempting to play down the impact of a compromised account, particularly one not connected to a practice's data storage, such as social media. Remember, however, that if you used a compromised account to promote your business, it may be connected to followers and clients; criminals can still use the opening to harm your reputation or look at private messages you have sent on the platform to clients. Always evaluate the potential impact of any account that is compromised and refer back to your data privacy and other legislation when you do.

Further learning

It is not important to know all the ways a password can be cracked – there are many. However, as you are now an able cybersecurity researcher, if you are interested in knowing more about the methods hackers use, do a quick internet search for "how hackers crack passwords". There are a number of short videos online that can give you quick insight. You will see how simple it can be. Alternatively, search and read an article on the top ways hackers steal your password.

Early in the book, the SolarWinds attack was mentioned. Some of the media stories around a potential password breach in connection to this may be interesting optional reading for those readers starting to become interested in some of the topics of this chapter (Fung & Sands, 2021).

*

Multi-factor authentication and biometrics

MFA or 2FA requires that after putting in an initial password or login credential to log into something, the user has to confirm their login with a second or further factor or credential.

Due to the increased use of MFA by many banks, authorities and services on a compulsory basis, many people actually are using it in some form or another. Most email accounts, cloud services and some software providers also have the option to sign in using MFA/2FA. As a practitioner, it is prudent to use this where it is offered, at all times.

For ease of reference, the term MFA will be used in this book to cover both scenarios but to briefly explain the differences:

- 2FA – the user will only have to input two factors
- MFA – the provider can ask for more than two factors. This might occur if you trigger any risk markers they have set up (which can include logging in from a new location or a new device)

Examples of a second (or further) login factor:

- Confirming your login via an authentication app (such as Microsoft Authenticator, Duo)
- Code from a physical token fob
- Verification of identity over Bluetooth, near-field communication (NFC) or USB
- Memorable information or security questions
- Smartcards
- Input of a single-use access code sent by email
- Input of a single-use access code sent by SMS
- Digital signature

MFA can discourage criminals. It can still be breached but makes it harder for them (Australian Cyber Security Centre [ACSC], n.d.). It sets up another wall around the cyber fortress you are building around your practice.

The most important things to remember from this section:

- MFA is one of the best ways to secure anything you log into right now
- MFA involves two stages (at least) when you log in – an initial login stage and then a second alternative verification step

Action points

In the previous section, on passwords, you were asked (action point 2), to enable MFA where it was possible. If you did not do that, go back to accounts where you can enable MFA and do so. Waiting until you log in next is not optimal, as you may be in a hurry at that time. So, put time aside to do this.

Best practice is to apply MFA to anything you connect to over the internet (NCSC, 2018b) – including bank accounts, government sites, cloud storage – anything with sensitive data pertaining to your practice or yourself.

Going deeper

Anything you come across in the chapters that is of particular interest, take a break to research more on the topic and go a little deeper. Alternatively, make a note to look up later, when you want to continue reading. Sometimes, we have read a term before – for example, two factor authentication – but not really understood all about it. That's why terminology and explanations are provided in these pages, so that you will feel it is easier to find, read and absorb information going forward.

Similarly, anything you have found difficult to absorb, check if there is information on the same topic in another format – a short video, for instance. There are a series of 2- to 4-minute videos posted by the City of London Police (Cyber Griffin, n.d.) (https://cybergriffin.police.uk/videos) that cover some practical information on being safe online and some of the threats we will discuss in Chapters 5–7. Much of the advice will be relevant wherever you are resident in the world. Some security professionals also post videos demonstrating how they try to get back at scammers, which can show another view and give insight into how far criminals will sometimes go.

Mark's case – Part 3

Don't be like Mark

Now a few more pages have passed, it is time to conclude Mark's case. If required, re-read Part 1 (p. 14) and Part 2 (p. 38). Before you read this last part, have a look at the notes you made so far, then continue.

Unfortunately, the nice lady on the phone to Mark was not from tax. She was very helpful and took all his credit card information; a couple of weeks later, he had a bill for his card showing he had spent up to his limit. Mark was shocked when he opened the statement, as he had not used the card. When he noticed the transactions processed the day his card was maxed out, it started with a smaller payment of 300 pounds, then soon after two larger ones that went up to his credit limit. He remembered the payment of 300 pounds and his heart sank. In an instant, some puzzle pieces just slotted together. Checking the data to his phone calls, he confirmed he'd been scammed by the "tax" lady.

Mark was unlucky. His information online shows him as a small business owner. It was time for him to send in his taxes. He was tired; he thought tax was calling him because the spoofed number matched an entry in his phone. Mark didn't think that it was quite late in the day to get a phone call. He didn't think that he had never before been chased for payment over the phone. He had also, if he had thought about it at the time, never paid his taxes partially over the phone before.

The lady on the phone had convinced him to give a lot of information on his card to her. Looking back, he simply had been swept away with how helpful she was. The idea of someone solving his problem had just felt so good that he had not considered that it was an offer that was too good to be true. Mark was also distracted and didn't think twice about the fact that he had given her a number of SMS codes from his phone – codes he would only need if using the card himself to purchase something. The caller's story that they were to approve paying the bill to tax seemed real to him, and he had quickly just given them to her, skipping over reading the text of the SMS, which would have shown they were purchase alerts from his bank. Later, Mark realised he had often judged his friend who had almost signed up to be a Bitcoin millionaire in an hour. Now, he realised he had also fallen into a trap, just in a different way.

Mark's story introduces some of the elements that underlie scams. In Chapters 6 and 7 more of these that practitioners have faced are covered, along with some of the ways to react if you find yourself a victim of cyber-enabled fraud.

Red flags

There are many red flags for all kinds of criminal activity. Throughout this book, focus will be on those that will start you thinking more broadly:

- Are you expecting the correspondence?
- Do you normally get an email, SMS, call from this place?
- Is the person's tone on the other side of the call/discussion (or tone of their written correspondence), different from what you would expect from the caller/company? Is there any variation in what you have experienced from them in the past?
- Are you being put under pressure? (Note, today, criminals know that this is widely written as a red flag, so some are learning to be more tempered with their pressure pace.)
- Are you being asked for personal information that the caller/corresponding party should have if they genuinely are who they say they are?
- Are you being asked to provide anything that pertains to your access to an account?

Triple check everything. Look for mistakes in the email address of the sender, the signature on the email and be careful about anything you are going to click on. If still in doubt, call the company.

In calling a company, never use the number written on something you have suspicions about, and do not call back the number a suspicious caller gives you. Look up a number on a past invoice, bill, statement, paperwork from the company claiming to call, and if you do not have one of those, look for a trusted website and find the contact numbers that way.

If any caller to you resists/pushes back when you say you will return their call later, this is a red flag, along with if they suggest an alternative phone number to reach them on. It's ok to note the number and play along that you will use it – just don't use it (except in any eventual report if it turns out to be attempted fraud – it might help protect others). Do your research as mentioned, and only call back a trusted number that you find and verify matches the company the caller said they are calling from.

Further reading

For the country you live in, you can check your government websites for examples of tax scams they currently are getting alerts of.

Similarly, some governments do publish information on how to be safe online in dealing with government and tax authorities (Example: GovUK, 2007). So, check for this advice too.

Spoofing:

Examples of resources on spoofing:

Federal Communications Commission (2021) have a website page on spoofing that they keep updated: https://www.fcc.gov/spoofing

---

Reminders:

Always listen to your instincts.

Never ignore a red flag.

Remember that like Mark, at the right time, place and given the "right" scenario, anyone is vulnerable to a cybercriminal's story.

Website

Just a short reminder that if you run a website for your practice, look into its security. Securing websites depends on where you host, publish, build or otherwise situate and run your site. The best advice will come from looking up the providers you use and potentially working with a relevant web professional.

Many practitioners set up a website or have someone design one that they run afterwards. This is fine but be aware to set up some security around the website. If you use a website-building tool that takes much of the design out of your hands, the security of the site may not be very visible, and you may need to look more deeply into how it is protected. If you largely run a site yourself, ensure to add a security tool around it. You will within, no time, see the number of breach attempts made on your site daily, and be shocked.

Third parties, mentioned earlier, are also where cyber risks can come in. Some third-party plug-ins and other additions to a website can bring vulnerabilities

(Lakshmanan, 2021), as can the website platform you use. Bear in mind that if you collect customer information, or sell anything via a website, you need to take extra care with the security of the site. A hacked website can affect your reputation and lead to business downtime and financial loss.

Distraction

One of the points with Mark's case, and why it is one of the case studies, is that it provides an idea of how, as practitioners, we will be approached by criminals who are looking to exploit weaknesses related to our roles or our business structures. Many practitioners – like Mark – may be running a smaller practice, working from a home office space, juggling sessions, accounting and administrative tasks.

It's worth remembering that a criminal will target a number of people, knowing that the precise MO they are following will, at some point, fit precisely with the timing, situation and context of the person they call. For example, a call from tax might not be seen as fully out of the ordinary, especially if the timing of the call fits with certain filings being due.

If Mark had been in contact with his accountant and more involved with his own paperwork, he may have been more aware to check details before handing over payment information. If he had been fully focused and not mixing home and work tasks, he might have been more alert to the red flags around him on paying a "deposit" to tax without any paperwork. He might have realised something was not quite right.

Through the pages until this point, we have looked at topics such as device security and the vulnerabilities of home offices. We have also looked at insecure networks (which can lead to data security issues) and the impact of a lack of cybersecurity awareness across all aspects of setting up to work online. Mark provides an example of a very different vulnerability in the home space – the human. When operating your home and work life in the same space, on the same equipment, you just may be more vulnerable to an attack (Okereafor & Manny, 2020). For example, a large percentage of cyberattacks are delivered by email. How discerning are you when switching from using devices for work to home purposes or when surrounded by distractions such as family life and obligations?

Being mindful of the potentiality of distraction in leading us to make a hasty and incorrect decision can be extremely valuable.

- Don't make a decision when you are distracted or juggling a number of things and an unexpected caller or email is pressuring you to do something out of the ordinary
- When receiving a call or an email and there being any requirement from it to provide information – personal, sensitive, banking or otherwise – always hesitate and think a little bit deeper about the request

• Standing back and taking time to review anything unusual carefully is a valuable part of the response toolkit for a practitioner. This message will be repeated through this book in different ways, and the different case studies provide you with the opportunity to fine-tune your new awareness skills and red flag–spotting abilities, as the information builds up through the chapters

---

Activity

Open your reflective notes – this will take five minutes.

1. Note how operating as a practitioner in a home–work mixed environment may impact your practice from a cybersecurity point of view
2. What will you remember to be more mindful to do if you are called with an unusual request and are busy, pressurised or distracted from focusing on clarifying what the request is before responding to it in any way?

A reminder that the simple reflective activities are part of your knowledge journey, and will ensure that not only will your practice and client data be immediately more secure but also that you activate positive behaviours and practices towards an ongoing secure pathway.

Case study break – Adrian

It is time to look at your first full case study. This one builds on some of the knowledge so far and will enable you to practise your reaction to the information given as the story unfolds.

When you look up the case study, try not to be tempted to read the others in the same section yet. Wait until you see instructions in the chapters to go to them, as you will get more out of them if you take them one-by-one after some of the knowledge has unfolded. The case studies are set up to give you opportunities to tune your cyberthreat radar. They cover areas covered by the book up to that point and also new territory that may come up in later chapters.

Turn to the back of the book and look up "The Full Case of Adrian" (p. 167). Read it slowly, step-by-step, adding to your reflective notes as you do. Take time to enjoy the reflective element of how your thoughts evolve as you read the sections – this can reveal how you have built your skills and resources when you do.

*

Securing other devices on a home network

It isn't just computers, phones and tablets that create cyber vulnerabilities on a home network. Other devices in our homes are both capturing data and are online, connected to our networks. Your household may use a considerable number of "smart" or internet-linked devices. Anything that connects online is a way in for a criminal. The various devices we have in our homes, along with their users, are argued by some as potentially "the weakest link in any IT security chain" (Abdullahi, 2015, p. 229). This is because we often do not think beyond setting up a device and using it. A network you use to connect any device you use in your practice, with client data on it, is a network you need to pay attention to, along with all the other devices connected to it.

The following devices and products are relevant here:

- Smart devices, such as the heating or electronic lighting you activate over Bluetooth or an app, e-readers, fitness gadgets, security cameras (including nanny cams), doorbells
- Smart white goods products connected to your network
- TVs, games consoles in use in your home on your network
- Any other device that can be connected online, including those of other users in your home that are on the network to which your practice devices are connected

Updates are as equally important for these products as for those you tradition-ally associate with security and your business tools (computer, OS, software as covered in the last chapter). Any reputable device connected to the internet will produce new versions and updates periodically, and ensuring you implement these updates is vitally important (Hattar, 2022).

There have been breaches of many smart home products (Abdullahi, 2015); this book will not name any specific cases as it can look as if a product is being singled out. The reality is any brand or product is vulnerable to a determined criminal. The problem is similar to that clarified in the last section: if any manufacturer fails to mitigate threats as they come, or to keep their security up to date, then that product might become your weakest link.

Some starter tips to mitigate the risks around any device linked to your network:

- Always change any default user IDs, passwords when installing a device. Use a unique, strong password on the device, and if it offers 2FA/MFA, enable it
- Connect devices to a fully secure internet router
- Keep what you allow the device to do (permissions) to a minimum of what is needed to run it, for example, if your kettle, that you can turn on via an app, is asking for permission to use your contacts and your photo gallery, don't enable this. (And you may want to review the product as to why it is asking for permissions beyond its scope of use!)

- Verify what information and data a device says it will store and why it is doing so, before activating it or the relevant settings
- Once activated, it can be wise to periodically check what data a device is storing – actively and passively. Sometimes, updates come or new terms and conditions; read them, don't just click "accept"
- Ensure before buying any device that it is security verified – along with checking for any reports of security breaches of the product, for example, if you buy a nanny cam, thoroughly review its own security, how frequently the company updates it and check reviews and vulnerabilities reported on the manufacturer
- Do read the manual – it may give other ideas on security you can enable for the product
- For devices that precisely have a purpose that you can access them outside the home via a mobile device, do take care. Mobile devices often have less security than a computer, so make sure you have robust security software on them and never connect to any of your home devices remotely from an insecure internet connection or public Wi-Fi
- Run device and software updates as soon as they are available
- Be wary of devices that never have updates, particularly ones you have had a while – nothing is that secure! Every device needs updates. Re-review the product
- Research for any other security best practices that would be pertinent for the devices you have

A short reflexive exercise with some examples that might help how you look at evaluating what a product/device can do:

On a practice level

- If product X needs to access data on your device, what exactly could someone manipulating the product extract from that?
- If product Y has not updated for some time and has now issued 3 new versions since you bought yours, are they still providing security updates for the version of the product you hold? If not, re-evaluate your use of the device
- Has anyone breached the products you use, in the past? What does the product have in place to ensure security today (research online)?

On a personal level

- While you check your devices for security bearing in mind your practice and clients, you are also ensuring that your personal data and your home are also secure

Personal assistants/virtual assistants

If you use a personal assistant/virtual assistant, such as Alexa, Google Assistant, Cortana or Siri, you need also to check that the device or software assistant you use is not active and passively attentive to conversations in the rooms you hold sessions with clients, including online sessions. Are your virtual assistants set to listen? These products have been hacked (Chung et al., 2017), and there are reports of them activating information they have heard, so ensuring that they are disabled when you are in client conversations is important. Even better is not enabling them on any devices used for client conversations (if online) and keeping them fully out of the room (if devices).

*

Second-hand devices and disposing of devices

This section returns to focusing on the main devices you might use in your practice (computers, tablets and phones) and the risks of using older and second-hand devices.

Older devices

While it can feel like an achievement to still be using a tablet from 2015, using older devices also comes with the same security risks as noted previously for older OSs and software. Older devices may not be receiving security updates or have the attention of their manufacturers making them more vulnerable to hackers. Which? show that it can vary from manufacturer to manufacturer how long they will issue security updates for older models of products. They recommend checking the manufacturer's security pages to find out whether an older device is still covered (Muyanja, 2020).

Action points

If you frequently change your devices, these points may not be so pertinent. However, if you tend to use something until it falls apart, then they will be important:

1. Review all devices you use to store confidential information. Check the model on the manufacturer's website – is the product still receiving security updates periodically?
2. For devices up to 2 years old, review annually. For devices over 2 years of age, review every six months. For devices over 4 years old, double-check whether the device is really still covered. Use the manufacturer's website and any research on the brand to gauge how long the device might be supported, so that you can start planning when to buy a replacement
3. You can also consider making an internet monitoring alert ("Google alert") for articles pertaining to disabling of support/security updates for your device(s)

or any other topics so far covered in this book, if you feel this may help to prompt you or get you on track

Second-hand devices

One thing that comes with being more cyber-aware is that media posts on cyber-security issues or threats become easier to digest. At certain times of the year, some particular articles are circulated or re-circulated. A couple of examples to highlight – Singles Day, Black Friday and Cyber Monday shopping events in November generate reminders around many issues connected to secure shopping, including alerts around fraudulent sites and card fraud. Christmas, similarly, high-lights the same topics alongside alerts related to charity scams, which escalate in holiday periods where there is often a little more active campaigning for funds – unfortunately, including from fraudsters.

Another thing brought up in the end-of-year festive period is the risk of second-hand devices (NCSC, 2020b). Electronic devices are becoming increasingly com-plex, and as a result, often more expensive. The second-hand market for them is attractive – it makes it possible to buy a higher-end device or newer model for a reduced price. Additionally, the recycling incentive is also clear.

As a practitioner handling sensitive data, it is important to inform yourself on the following when considering purchasing a second-hand device:

1. Buy a second-hand device only from a reputable source. This is not a guaran-tee (you are still vulnerable to the integrity of the people working there), but it is safer than buying from a non-reputable source
2. Inform yourself on how the device has been reset and cleaned for a new user. If you are buying from a second-hand retailer, ask them or read up on their policies of how they prepare devices for customers. This will give you an idea of whether the retailer is ensuring that the devices they sell are secure. If there is nothing written on how they make devices safe, it is likely they only perform factory resets and do not scan products they have purchased for threats such as malware, which can remain on a device even after a full reinstall
3. Even if your device has been reset, you should do your own factory reset prior to using it (NCSC, 2020c). If you do not know how to, ask someone you trust to do it
4. Check the impact of the age of the second-hand device. Remember that newer models may have their software and security more frequently updated than older models. In 2020, Which? published an article about why some second-hand phones could be a security risk, indicating that around 31% of second-hand mobile phone sales at some popular retailers were models no longer receiving manufacturer security updates (Muyanja, 2020)
5. An alternative to recycling, if you are keen to reduce the environmental impact, is to look for eco-friendly devices. The effort some brands put into the following is often overlooked: using recycled materials, non-toxic

materials, more eco-friendly materials where possible; creating efficient devices with lower energy usage and ensuring devices can be recycled after use and have lower emission and radiation levels (Eco Friend, n.d.). A newer device made of recyclable materials and that uses less energy and produces less radiation will still keep you on track to reducing your eco-footprint, and at the same time, ensure more security around your client data and interactions

Selling devices

Again, as much as recycling is a salient topic, if you decide to sell a device (computer, tablet, phone or other) you have used in connection with your practice, then you should be aware it is difficult to remove all traces of data fully from devices. It is important you make an informed decision if you decide to sell rather than fully, physically destroy a device (CISA, 2021).

Some advice if you do go ahead with selling a device:

1. Ensure you sanitise the device prior to the sale. A factory reset is not enough. Involve a qualified IT professional, as needed, and inform yourself fully on the risks (CISA, 2021; NCSC, 2020d)
2. Reflect on how sensitive the data is that has been stored on the device towards your decision to sell it
3. If selling via a retailer, point 1 still applies. You do still need to pursue performing full erasure and reset prior to passing to them. If you do not, you are leaving data up for discovery in the wrong hands

Safe disposal of a device

Currently, the best way to prevent anyone retrieving any traces of information from a device is to physically destroy any part of the device that can store data (CISA, 2021). It is recommended that you do this prior to putting a device in the bin or taking it to a recycling point. If you are determined to sanitise the product instead of destroying it, then apply the advice from point 1 of the last section.

The NCSC (2020b) also provides lists of devices that have storage but are not always automatically considered (e.g. printers); prior to sale or disposal, these also need evaluation as to whether they have storage capabilities.

Note that if you have a device that is defective, it does not mean that data stored cannot be accessed if the device is fixed or the hard drive or other storage media is moved to another device; research how to destroy or sanitise any part of a defective device prior to disposal (NCSC, 2020b).

Larger companies

Devices from larger companies with a large volume of data particularly should take advice from a professional and use certified products for any erasure.

Passing a device to a member of the family

While tempting to recycle by passing a device to a family member, reflect on the information provided so far and evaluate if this is the right action to take. The same due care to sanitise the device must be taken if you decide to do this (CISA, 2021). Perform research for the relevant device.

Data retention for record purposes

Before erasing any device, whether prior to sale or destruction, ensure any records you are obliged to keep as a practitioner are safely transferred to a new, secure device.

Non-supported devices

If you, despite all the advice in this chapter (and book), buy and determine to use in your practice a device, product or software that no longer is supported by its manufacturer and is obsolete, you should understand you are putting your clients at risk. Remember the news stories in the first chapter. A data breach (and even just the perception of it) can have lasting consequences for clients. Revert to the guidelines, ethics, legislation you are required to follow for your profession. If this was still not enough to deter you, as a minimum please at least research how to mitigate some of the risks (NCSC, 2020a).

Further reading

Something this time for those of you who are more technical. https://tweaks.com/ (Tweaks, n.d.) is a website run by Advanced PC Media LLC, which develops software for the Microsoft Windows platform. On this site, various "tweaks" are available for older and newer Windows systems. If you use a Windows system and have an affinity for technology, you might find their pages interesting. Tweaks on an OS are the small things that can be done to optimise it, so they have tips on security, performance, usability and more.

Summary

Among other topics, this chapter has covered the following:

- Looked at some of the vulnerabilities of a home office or a network set up by a practitioner themselves (as opposed to an IT security team that might be found in a corporation)
- Discussed the vulnerability of second-hand and older devices
- Reviewed the importance of using complex passwords and MFA
- Concluded a case study that shows the importance of pausing to think about a request and double-checking whether it is legitimate

A lot has been achieved in these first chapters. With the information and activities so far, you have now, among other things, achieved the following:

- Understanding of why cybersecurity is vital to protect your practice and customers
- Gained knowledge of some cyber terms
- Checked the security of your devices
- Started to learn about spotting red flags
- Looked at network, router and device security
- Evaluated and set up secure passwords/passphrases where needed
- Enabled MFA where you are able
- Started building a new understanding of how to practically implement the data security noted in the legislation and ethics guidelines practitioners adhere to

References

Abdullahi, A. (2015). Cyber security challenges within the connected home ecosystem futures. *Procedia Computer Science, 61,* 227–232. https://doi.org/10.1016/j.procs.2015.09.201

Australian Cyber Security Centre. (n.d.). *Multi-factor authentication.* Australian Government. https://www.cyber.gov.au/mfa

Chung, H., Iorga, M., Voas, J., & Lee, S. (2017). Alexa, can I trust you? *Computer, 50*(9), 100–104. https://doi.org/10.1109/MC.2017.3571053

CISA. (2021, February 1). *Security tip (ST18-005) proper disposal of electronic devices.* https://www.cisa.gov/tips/st18-005

CIRT. (2021). *Default passwords.* https://cirt.net/passwords

Delaney, J. R. (2021, December 13). *The best wireless routers for 2022.* PC Mag. https://uk.pcmag.com/routers/8151/the-best-wireless-routers

Eco Friend. (n.d.). *8 most eco-friendly mobile phones ever manufactured.* https://ecofriend.org/8-most-eco-friendly-mobile-phones-ever-manufactured/

FBI. (n.d.). *Protected voices: Passphrases and multi-factor authentication.* https://www.fbi.gov/video-repository/protected-voices-passphrases-and-mfa-102319.mp4/view

Federal Communications Commission. (2021). *Caller ID spoofing.* https://www.fcc.gov/spoofing

Fung, B., & Sands, G. (2021, February 26). *Former SolarWinds CEO blames intern for "solarwinds123" password leak.* CNN Politics. https://edition.cnn.com/2021/02/26/politics/solarwinds123-password-intern/index.html

Goodin, D. (2020, June 9). *Mystery malware steals 26M passwords from 3M PCs: Are you affected?* Ars Technica. https://arstechnica.com/gadgets/2021/06/nameless-malware-collects-1-2tb-of-sensitive-data-and-stashes-it-online/

GovUK. (2007, February 5). *How HM revenue and customs keeps you safe online.* Crown Copyright. https://www.gov.uk/government/publications/how-hm-revenue-and-customs-keeps-you-safe-online

Hattar, M. (2022, January 3). *IoT's importance is growing rapidly, but its security is still weak.* SecurityWeek. https://www.securityweek.com/iots-importance-growing-rapidly-its-security-still-weak

Hoffman, C. (2017, July 3). *How to find your router's IP address on any computer, smartphone, or tablet*. How-to-Geek. https://www.howtogeek.com/233952/how-to-find-your-routers-ip-address-on-any-computer-smartphone-or-tablet/

Krebs, B. (n.d.). *Password do's and don'ts*. Krebs on Security. https://krebsonsecurity.com/password-dos-and-donts/

Lakshmanan, R. (2021, March 17). *Flaws in two popular wordpress plugins affect over 7 million websites*. The Hacker News. https://thehackernews.com/2021/03/flaws-in-two-popular-wordpress-plugins.html

Laughlin, A. (2021, June 9). *Best password managers*. Which? https://www.which.co.uk/reviews/antivirus-software-packages/article/best-password-managers-a3EGi5s8WIvU

Muyanja, L. (2020, July 31). *Why some second-hand phones could be a security risk*. Which? https://www.which.co.uk/news/2020/07/mobile-phones-recycling-and-security/

National Cyber Security Centre. (2018a, November 19). *Password administration for system owners*. Crown Copyright. https://www.ncsc.gov.uk/collection/passwords/password-manager-buyers-guide

National Cyber Security Centre. (2018b, December 3). *Multi-factor authentication for online services*. Crown Copyright. https://www.ncsc.gov.uk/guidance/multi-factor-authentication-online-services

National Cyber Security Centre. (2019a, April 21). *Passwords, passwords everywhere*. Crown Copyright. https://www.ncsc.gov.uk/blog-post/passwords-passwords-everywhere

National Cyber Security Centre. (2019b, April 21). *Protected voices: Most hacked passwords revealed as UK cyber survey exposes gaps in online security*. Crown Copyright. https://www.ncsc.gov.uk/news/most-hacked-passwords-revealed-as-uk-cyber-survey-exposes-gaps-in-online-security

National Cyber Security Centre. (2020a, January 22). *Mobile device guidance*. Crown Copyright. https://www.ncsc.gov.uk/collection/mobile-device-guidance/managing-the-risks-from-obsolete-products

National Cyber Security Centre. (2020b, February 13). *Secure sanitisation of storage media*. Crown Copyright. https://www.ncsc.gov.uk/guidance/secure-sanitisation-storage-media

National Cyber Security Centre. (2020c, December 28). *Buying and selling second-hand devices*. Crown Copyright. https://www.ncsc.gov.uk/guidance/buying-selling-second-hand-devices

National Cyber Security Centre. (2020d, December 28). *Erasing personal data from second-hand devices*. Crown Copyright. https://www.ncsc.gov.uk/blog-post/erasing-personal-data-second-hand-devices

National Institute of Standards and Technology. (2017). *NIST special publication 800–63B digital identity guidelines*. https://pages.nist.gov/800-63-3/sp800-63b.html

Norton, K. (2022). Wi-Fi. In *Webopedia*. https://www.webopedia.com/definitions/wi-fi/

Okereafor, K., & Manny, P. (2020). Understanding cybersecurity challenges of telecommuting and video conferencing applications in the Covid-19 pandemic. *International Journal in IT & Engineering, 8*(6), 13–23. http://doi.org/10.6084/m9.figshare.12421049

Security.org. (n.d.). *How secure is my password?* https://www.security.org/how-secure-is-my-password/

Tung, L. (2021, June 14). *This data and password-stealing malware is spreading in an unusual way*. ZDNet. https://www.zdnet.com/article/this-data-and-password-stealing-malware-is-spreading-in-an-unusual-way/

Tweaks. (n.d.). *Microsoft windows tweaks, tips and how-to articles*. https://tweaks.com/

Use a Passphrase. (n.d.). https://www.useapassphrase.com/

Wakefield, J. (2021, May 6). *Millions at security risk from old routers, Which? warns*. BBC News. https://www.bbc.com/news/technology-56996717

Chapter 4

Keeping communications confidential

Introduction

The rise in people working from home and new attention to exploiting the tools they use has positively led to more awareness on the security flaws of communications tools. Articles and news stories showed criminals honing their skills; they colourfully described meetings being "bombed" by criminals causing mischief (Zoombombing, 2021). What perhaps was less covered is that criminals have, for a very long time, been infiltrating calls invisibly. They also sell on the darknet what they find out, along with hacked account credentials, or even give them away for free (Mathews, 2020).

Everyone providing a service is looking to create a good customer experience for their clients. In today's age, the use of new technological tools and advances can help facilitate that. New tools come with new risks, however, for industries such as healthcare in ensuring data and client privacy (Lustgarten et al., 2020). Cybercriminals will also continue to be interested in "targeting vulnerable people and systems" (Pranggono & Arabo, 2020, p. 1), so ways of operating our tools and our own responses and cyber competences simply have to be strengthened, including when using communications tools.

Regarding terminology, the chapter uses the terms video conferencing, online conferencing/communications tools and other terms that essentially (unless otherwise specified) cover any product that enables video, audio or typed conversations:

- with another person or group of people
- with this conversation occurring with or without a camera enabled
- via the internet or via a mobile network

Please don't skip this chapter if you only work with clients face-to-face as the advice provided is relevant for practitioners using conferencing tools on any device (phone, tablet, PC) to do any of the following:

- Talk or write to clients
- Undergo supervision

DOI: 10.4324/9781003184805-5

- Join meetings with groups, accreditation bodies, societies or any other where professional information is shared
- Hold any form of meeting or chat conversation with peers

More will be covered later on how in general practitioners should take great care about what they add in large "chat" groups with no membership screening, controls and deletion rules.

Don't feel alarmed by the contents of this chapter. The actions of securing your network, router and logins in the previous chapter all add layers towards preventing someone accessing a session on a communications tool (Okereafor & Manny, 2020). This chapter, however, connects more deeply to the topics of choosing secure tools and using the features they have. It also connects to how we need to make ethical, informed decisions around the security of the spaces where we share information online. The advice will help inform what you should think about and when to ensure or insist on better security and controls in an online space. Additionally, many of you likely use communications tools beyond your practice, so this information will have double use.

The chapter will build and improve:

Awareness

of how to check whether the communications tools you use are secure

Understanding

of what you expose both yourself and your clients to if you do not use a reliable tool

Information security practices

through new reflective and applied approaches to protecting your clients' data in online communications

*

Vulnerabilities

This section will address the vulnerabilities around communications tools currently most relevant to practitioners operating in confidential spaces. This enables insight into the importance of making best-practice decisions on which communication tools to use.

Why are these tools interesting to criminals?

For a cybercriminal, online meetings and communications tools are goldmines for obtaining/exposing secret, classified and confidential information.

Man-in-the-middle attacks

This is when an attacker either gains entry to a call or accesses its recording, if there is one (Okereafor & Manny, 2020). It is useful at this stage to learn the difference between passive and active attacks. Passive attacks occur in the background and may not fully impact the system/device/software being breached, meaning the user may still be able to operate unaware that someone is listening in or gathering information. Active attacks have, as implied, a more visible impact: something will be changed or transmitted, and the system may be disabled or become non-functional.

A passive attack on a communication tool would be someone reading chats or snooping on a call undetected. An attack can start passively and then become more active, if the attacker decides to become visible after being in the background. Alternatively, in a call with a large number of participants, an attacker may go undetected – and even participate with the other practitioners. These threats apply to browser based tools and apps and written chat conversations are also infiltrated.

Zoombombing, which we covered earlier (possible on any video conferencing tool), is a type of man-in-the-middle attack, with a disrupter jumping into online video calls out of nowhere (Zoombombing, 2021). Most of these incursions are purely to cause mischief. However, many of them have occurred in arenas such as online teaching, webinars, work meetings. So, in meetings where the disruption also comes with a breach of privacy and uncertainty as to what the intruder has been listening to.

Man-in-the-middle attacks can occur due to malware being on your computer/ device or someone accessing it via an insecure router. This is why the defences you have put in place so far are important, as well as the tips that will come later in the chapter around securing your use of communications tools.

Malware transmission

Be aware that fake installations of a communications product or fake updates sometimes circulate that turn out to be malware. Always check what you are installing, don't click on anything unexpected (check the apps checklist at the back of this book).
Beware also of links or files posted by someone you don't know in the chat field of a call or in a chat discussion. Attackers joining calls or chat groups have used this as a way to proliferate malware. Monitoring activity is easier when you are in a 1:1 conversation than in a larger audience call, where multiple people may be posting, and participants may not think twice before clicking on something.

Choices

The actions coming in the next section involve reviewing what you use today. As noted in the first chapters of this book, reviewing the products you use on a regular basis, as a practitioner operating with confidential information, is vital. You may have may fallen into a comfort zone with your communications tools, using the same ones as you have for years or just accepting one your peers use, or a group you have joined is utilising. To secure the data in your practice, you need to more actively ensure you are using secure tools. Pay attention also to media alerts about communications tools, they can provide up-to-date information about their vulnerabilities and risks.

There is a very real risk of exposure for clients if you use a tool with inadequate security. A criminal attempting to breach software will keep looking for the ways in, and once they find them, others will join using the same hole in security. A reliable software provider will react quickly, fixing the vulnerability and leaving the criminals to go find the next one. This is why using the most secure products is recommended.

Using free conferencing tools

Free versions of online conferencing/chat tools may come with less security and hosting controls, making it pertinent to research what you are using. Because you handle confidential data, you need to always check if using a free version of a product means less security than a paid or subscription version. If the difference between free and paid is how many background colours you can pick from, that is a whole other thing. It is security that is the area not up for compromise!

Myth busting

A little of some of the motivation for this book emerged with spotting the following written by practitioners online:

I read in the news they fixed the bug; it is safe now and fine

If you read a headline that a communications app/tool has fixed a privacy issue or a security issue – still do your own research as to the overall security of the app/tool and suitability to use it with clients.

It's ok, it has encryption

Encryption, for criminals, is more of a hurdle than a barrier. Eventually, any form of it can be broken. The most secure communications tools have been breached (Barrett, 2021), and authorities themselves have both infiltrated apps and set them up to find criminal networks (Europol, 2021).

The product is safe, it's GDPR compliant

A product saying it is General Data Protection Regulation (GDPR) compliant (or compliant with any other data privacy law) does not make it data secure. It means it has fulfilled criteria towards being compliant with the legislation and may offer functionality that will help the user with aspects of GDPR/other, such as deletion, data storage/processing capabilities. It does not mean that the product cannot be breached, infiltrated, hacked or compromised in any way. To protect the product, you still need cybersecurity around it and around your use of it. Being compliant with legislation is not synonymous with having secure controls around your use of the cyberspace.

I'm not sharing any names (regarding sharing client stories in large chat groups with no regulation)

In an experiment, the author joined a forum for a large group of practitioners with a fake name, fake photo created by a deepfake AI generator, and an email address created in five minutes. After joining different groups, it was possible to read everything posted without anyone asking questions as to who the new member in the group was.

The conversations included chat about particular client scenarios the practitioners wanted advice on, handling clients, contracts and other aspects that come up on a daily basis. The group was set up with only the best intentions of sharing and community, but from it, someone lurking and gaining information (like in this experiment) could go on to publish a lot of information about clients, along with the name and contact of their practitioners.

Practitioners should not be in any online discussion or chat group asking for advice on dealing with clients or sharing information on clients, where the group has no membership screening, controls and deletion rules. Every conversation you have or message you send is transmitted to the device of everyone else in that conversation, leaving that transmission not just vulnerable to what happens on your device and use of software but also everyone else's in that conversation.

You do need to know precisely who is in those conversations/discussions, whether they are applying cybersecure practices and how they are deleting any messages or recordings. Every person in a group share should be an active, known member. Also, whereas you may have informed your clients you may bring up their case in the supervision, have you informed them you might bring them up in an unregulated peer group? Every client must have the chance to agree/disagree up-front whether you can share information about them in such a setting and the client should be aware of the risks of transmission of data or conversations in the cyberspace. Changing names is not enough, you still need permission to share a story that has been told to you confidentially and to expose that information.

If you still have doubts as to why the points in this section have been made, read articles on the Vastaamo case in Finland. Particularly, the Wired articles by Ralston depict how it can feel for someone afraid their innermost secrets have been exposed – even if they are not sure their records will end up seen by people close to them or that their name will be linked to what is exposed (Ralston, 2020, 2021).

Always remember also that many messaging tools have not been built for the purposes of exchanging confidential data. They have been built to enable communication and to service a huge audience of users. That said, communications tools and apps don't want to hit the news due to questionable security, and reputable products will patch their security relatively quickly. This does not mean that another security risk will never come along. At this point, many conferencing tools and apps have been questioned for their data policies. Remember then the value of doing regular research on the tools you use. While manufacturers need to ensure product security, it will always remain the responsibility of anyone signing up to use a product to know it and use it securely and responsibly.

The next section will move onto action points towards establishing solid new behaviours and best practices for the secure use of the communications tools you decide to use in your practice.

Action points

Check your tools

Action 1

Perform an online search on the security for each video conferencing tool, chat tool, communications software/app you use today.

Search: "Is XYZ cybersecure" – replace XYZ with the tool you use.

Look for search results from the following:

- Reputable technology websites/magazines
- Security websites/magazines
- Newspapers

- Filter to articles from the last 3–6 months; widen search to longer periods if you need to, after that
- Check the product's own information too – how much does it reveal about what the manufacturer does to improve its security?
- Evaluate if you are happy to continue using the tool you have researched

Action 2

Research for best-in-class products to switch to or consider, try searching for the following:

- "What is the most secure video conferencing software in 20XX"? Replace XX with the correct year. Replace video conferencing with the term that best narrows down what you are researching (Examples: conferencing software, chat apps or communications tools)

Action 3

Review if you are optimally using all the security features that your product offers.

Action 4

Put on your calendar a recurring reminder to once a year re-check to find out whether the video conferencing tools you use are the safest options to use with your clients (and even privately).

Tips for performing annual reviews:

Look for stories on attacks on your product ("cyberattacks + XYZ product" or "vulnerabilities found + XYZ product") since your last review. Review the cyber issues the product has had in that period, and consider the following:

How responsive was the product to the issue(s)?
Have other products had the same issues?
Evaluate whether it is a product you can continue to use

Check for new features in your products that you haven't yet applied that will help with security around your calls

Use the security tools in the product

Similar to previous advice, if your video conferencing platform offers extra security functionality, take it. It may be there because a number of breaches or incidents have led to it being needed. Security features may include options on how to log in and how to allow people to join the meeting. Passwords, 2FA, waiting room/ lobby controls may seem like friction to the experience of joining a meeting, but they are often there because something has happened before. In the previous chapter we paused to reflect on how the increased complexity of passwords has come with a sense of increased friction, but on balance how this is now unavoidable; it is the same here. When most communications tools emerged, users just signed up and were good to go. There was very little use of passwords to gain access to a meeting, and there was little by way of encryption and extra layers of security. Take a pause to recognise that those days are gone; to be able to use new, evolving technology to service clients, we also need to apply security measures (Lustgarten et al., 2020). It is what it is: with one comes the other. Being more digital needs to be seen as going hand-in-hand with being more cybersecure.

Reminders for every practitioner

Remember security is multi-layered, so a secure device, network, good
credentials all build up as being a part of this, but communications tools
are another door in; – therefore, the advice in this chapter is important.
Some reminders to be clear on, connected to previous advice:

- Don't postpone updates of your devices, software, tools and apps.
  Run them as soon as you see them; remember, they are there for a
  reason
- Always evaluate the audience and security before you share something
  over the cyberspace pertaining to a confidential data set, – whether in
  conversation, by chat, by email or other transmission.
- Don't forget communications tools apply to all devices – phone,
  tablet, computer
- Any communications tool or software needs periodic review
- If you use your devices personally and with clients, you need to
  evaluate all communications tools on them equally. Don't assume
  you can "just" use less secure apps with friends and family. Less
  safe apps will provide criminals a way into your device
- *Never* communicate with clients over an insecure network

In Chapter 8 we will look more closely at the importance of discussing
with your client how you are interacting using online tools and ensuring
disclosure of the risks and your client's understanding of the risks.

Importance of periodic re-checks

Just a brief recap on why, for some of the activities in this book, you have now
scheduled an annual review:

- Software gets old – things can change quickly, and the most secure product
  can be overtaken by another that may offer more coverage or features for
  similar pricing
- When software companies do not update their products, the products become
  more susceptible to breaches. It may only be in an annual review that you
  realise a product is not as strong as it used to be
- Conversely, sometimes when a product is upgraded, there can be errors and
  weaknesses in the new version that increase chances for hackers to get in.
  Criminals are always also looking for ways into both new and old versions of
  a product, and particularly products used by a lot of people. An active, evolving product will arguably match threats as they unfold

- Cybercriminals and fraudsters are always a step ahead of the game. Their methods evolve constantly. They are always looking to find a new way in, making it vital to review periodically that the product you use is keeping up with changing threat landscape.

*

Checklist: basics for using communications/ conferencing tools with clients

Know your product

Have you recently reviewed whether your product is secure and fit for your practice? Ensure you are updated to the latest version. Are you happy with the security controls it offers you for meetings, or is there a product that will give you more options?

Update

Run any updates as and when they come up for installation. Same for any updates to the device you will communicate from.

Password protect your calls

Be careful how you share your meeting IDs and always ensure to add a password if the discussion will have confidential information or be a confidential client conversation.

The host starts the call

If you have settings that the host must join before call starts, use this setting. This ensures you are clear about who has joined after you.

Waiting room

If there is a waiting room filter, this also makes sure no one joins until you can take a break from your conversation to check who it is. Use it!

Know your attendees

Check who has called in if their name or number is not one you recognise. If you do not have a waiting room function, you need to listen out or look for when someone new joins. If an unidentified caller does not respond to requests to identify themselves, take steps to remove them and not to continue any conversation until they are out of the call.

Keep to small groups

If you are talking about something confidential online and you have invited a lot of people, consider if you can ably monitor the audience members when they join. Consider splitting the call to smaller groups or have someone assist checking names during the call.

Meeting forward alerts

If you use a calendar-linked product, you may be able to set an alert where you can see if someone has forwarded your invitation. You can then review such alerts as to whether the forward is appropriate. If someone has been invited who should not have access to the information you will share in the call, take steps.

Recordings

If you are hosting something that includes confidential information or sharing information about clients, it is very strongly recommended that such meetings are not recorded. Data storage is not just on your side but on the side of those who have access to a recording. You might think that most platforms where you can upload a video recording for view by the public ensure that the video is "non-downloadable" – think again. There are various ways and tricks out there to breach controls and download content – some of which anyone can master.

Review terms and conditions

Check the privacy and data storage policy of the communications tools you use or are considering to use. Review the permissions and access to your device that they require you to allow.

*

Checklist: basics for using chat tools with clients

Know the risks

When you write something, this may be stored by you, your client and the software product/app you are using. This makes it unlikely you can ever use any chat product 100% securely. Therefore, if you are offering chat support to clients, you do need to consider at least the following factors carefully.

Know your product

Have you recently reviewed whether your product is secure and fit for your practice? Ensure you are updated to the latest version.

Encryption

Do you have a product that encrypts calls/chats? Is this feature enabled? Note that this does not make the product bullet-proof by any means, but it can help protect content from less seasoned criminals.

Contracting

If you agree or arrange to support your clients via SMS, email or chat in the time between appointments, ensure that they are aware of the risk of sharing information online.

Boundaries

Set the boundaries or limit of the content you feel is appropriate to be shared online with clients between appointments. Make this clear upfront.

Disclaimers

Ensure that you have implemented disclaimers or confirm in writing the risks with your client (in your contract or other).

Data privacy laws

Re-check and verify data privacy laws (including GDPR in your country if you are in Europe, or the equivalent legislation where you are) for expectations on data storage and deletion. How long should you retain chats/emails between you and your client? Make sure this is part of your contract. Remember also that many practitioners are expected to make notes on their sessions with clients and keep them; if you are having "chat sessions", review how you are transferring the information from them to your notes prior to deletion of the content in the chat tool.

Review terms and conditions

Check the privacy and data storage policy of the tools you use or are considering to use. Review the permissions and access to your device that they require you to allow.

Written coaching sessions

If you offer coaching sessions that are 100% in writing – over chat/email (rare, but some do) – you particularly need to consider how you and your client contract on how you both will store, retain and delete the data.

Jessica's dilemma

Jessica is in a peer student counselling group using a chat app she has added to her phone. Recently, some of her peers started sharing stories about clients to get feedback. At first, it was exciting seeing all the dilemmas and stories from other people's practices. Over time, however, more people were joining this group and more and more stories were being told. Jessica asked whether there are any rules for what is shared in the group, and requirements for those who are in it. She was told "No" and that it's just a nice, informal place for people to learn from each other.

Jessica now herself has a client with an issue she could use some help on. She really wants to support her client and knows that sharing the client's story in the group will get her some replies and thoughts from her peers.

Activity

Reflect on what Jessica should do.
What would you do?

Supervision, peer groups and webinars

Every time you share information either verbally or in writing over the cyberspace, it as at risk of being breached. Each person you share it with, increases the risk as you have no control over how they handle the information on their side, and how they are securing their devices. Information security is an important part of cybersecurity and it includes being cognisant of only sharing data that we have permission to share and sharing it securely. Most practitioners engage in supervision, peer practice groups and share knowledge in webinars or other fora. There are important considerations to make before sharing any client-related information in these spaces.

Supervision

Supervisors are trained in how to operate their sessions. However, the following are some points towards ensuring good cyber practices in any supervision arrangement.

Group supervision

- The group should ensure to use a secure conferencing tool if not meeting face-to-face
- The supervisor should ensure all participants are agreed on confidentiality, including taking care as to how any notes, logs, reflections are stored by individual practitioners
- Supervision groups should not share information on clients in written form or across email or any apps. If the group, however, still takes a decision to

do this (not advised), then all participants of the group should discuss a number of things first, including agreeing on the most secure way to do this and contracting in the group on deleting content on the sides of all recipients. Additionally, most practitioners inform their clients that they may discuss their case in a trusted space with a supervisor, but typically the implication is that they do so verbally. Therefore, any decision to share information in written form in a supervision group should be very clearly disclosed to clients in contracting. As covered previously, it is not enough that the names are changed, any data breach disclosed to a client will put them in a position of being fearful that their innermost world has been exposed

1:1 supervision

- Ensure you are talking to your supervisor on a secure conferencing tool if you are not meeting face-to-face
- Store any notes as securely as you would client session notes
- It is not advised to share anything in writing pertaining to clients over the cyberspace, but if you decide to do that, ensure that both you and your supervisor delete this information after a certain period of time

Peer practice groups

- Consider to, as a minimum, apply the points raised in the group supervision section.

Training and peer discussion/chat groups

These may include the following:

- Peer-practice groups
- Any other practitioner group discussions
- Webinars
- CPD training

Before anyone shares client-related information in any of these settings, really consider ethics. In nearly all cases it will *not* be appropriate that you share client-related information shared in confidence with you. If you still decide to, the following should be clear:

- Have you informed your client you will share information about them in such a setting? Again, anonymisation does not take this responsibility away!
- Do you know who is in your group, especially if a large group? Remember, you are sharing with each person listening or reading
- Has the group agreed on confidentiality around discussions?
- Has the group established clear boundaries and ground rules around the deletion of any written notes and/or recordings after a period of time? Remember, every time you share something you increase the risk of exposure of it by

the number of people you share it with. Every person who receives a copy of anything shared, their device/network/accounts – can be compromised

Unregulated chat groups and online forums

Sharing client information in unregulated chat groups or online forums should be a no-go for any and all practitioners.

"Ah, but it's just talk . . . and sharing to learn"

No, it is not. It is data about your client. It's personal information about the innermost world of your client, shared only with you, and they are not expecting it to be shared with multiple others unless you have contracted with them that you are going to do so. That contracting conversation should also openly inform the client of the increased risk of exposure of data where it is shared with multiple parties and the practitioner should actively seek their consent.

Setting parameters

Any group should have underlying written rules as to how client information, cases and data are shared. As a very minimum, all members should be known, active and confirm they have adequate security on their devices and will delete information on an agreed basis.

Verify the members periodically – look for unusual and fake names and know each of your members.

Inactive/dormant members should be removed

While it is friendly to accept that some people only want to be in the background of a group; their lack of participation means you cannot be sure if they are still who they say they are, and the account has not been taken over or transferred. Everyone in a group receiving information about your clients should have a purpose to do so and their identity should be crystal clear.

If you are still feeling lenient, how do you benefit from inactive members? Ultimately, all they serve is being another party that receives information on your client. Do you know how they are handling this? It will only take the breach of one of the devices you share information with, for your data to be taken by a criminal. So, with each person you share client data, cases or stories with, you increase your cyber-vulnerability footprint.

"Ah, but I change the name"

This has been covered but is a vitally important message. Put yourself in your clients' shoes. Would you feel OK that your information was being shared out there with people you do not know? How would you feel if your information was breached and read or heard by anyone who gained access to it – even with your name changed?

Activity

Open your reflective notes.
Read the following and note what you would do:

> You have booked a meeting you will host as a supervisor with a group
> of six supervisees. This will be held using conferencing software you
> have checked as secure. You send an invitation over secure mail with a
> link to the call and the password to dial in.

Just before the meeting, one of the participants sends a chat message to all
the participants. The message is sent over a popular phone chat application
that has been in the media before as having questionable data privacy. You
have been meaning to talk to them about their use of this app. The participant
asks for a copy of the meeting information. Another participant replies by
copying the full invitation link and password into the chat.

Jessica's solution

Revisit the notes you made on Jessica's dilemma. This is what Jessica decided
to do:

> Jessica really liked the shared stories in the large peer chat group, but something
> didn't feel right. After consulting the ethical guidelines for the professional body
> she referred to, and some soul searching, Jessica decided to leave the group.

Putting herself in the shoes of a client, she considered how she would feel if her
counsellor was sharing information with so many people without her knowing.
Jessica realised that even though client names were not mentioned, it felt like a
breach of trust and exposure, particularly as the group had no rules and just added
new members without verifying them. There were also many people in the group
with no group lead, so she was not sure where to take the discussion to form some
better practices.

Jessica signed up with a supervisor who worked with groups. That way she felt
she could still hear a variety of interesting scenarios and also take her own questions. This did feel right. It was a smaller, safe and trusted group that fully contracted on how they each handled the information they shared. Jessica ensured all
her clients knew she might take elements of her conversations to her supervision
sessions. She also explained that any identifying information about them was not
shared and that this was a trusted, safe group that only used a secure conferencing
tool for its sessions, which were not recorded.

Jessica was also comforted that her supervisor paid good attention to security, even on smaller points such as requesting all group participants not to share the links and passwords to calls over chat apps. The supervisor explained to them that criminals can passively attend calls in the background, and to help prevent this, they should only exchange meeting data over secure email.

Summary

Among other topics this chapter has covered the following:

- Unfolded some of the vulnerabilities of communications tools
- Highlighted the need to take responsibility for the tools you choose to use
- Clarified the importance of applying any security options available
- Demonstrated how to review products on a regular basis and provided action points to be concluded before moving to the next chapter
- Provided starter checklists on the basics towards ensuring better security around online meetings and using chat applications

You are now able to explain to your clients how you review the tools you use to communicate with them and the risks to their data.

Added to that, if you look back at your work so far on the action points in this book, you will now also be able to explain to clients how you protect your practice as best you can, through your choices and application of defences. This is arguably part of true ethical cyber practices for all practitioners.

References

Barrett, B. (2021, April 24). *Security news this week: Signal's founder hacked a notorious phone-cracking device*. Wired. https://www.wired.com/story/signal-cellebrite-hack-app-store-scams-security-news/

Europol. (2021, June 8). *800 criminals arrested in biggest ever law enforcement operation against encrypted communication*. https://www.europol.europa.eu/newsroom/news/800-criminals-arrested-in-biggest-ever-law-enforcement-operation-against-encrypted-communication

Lustgarten, S. D., Garrison, Y. L., Sinnard, M. T., & Flynn, A. W. (2020). Digital privacy in mental healthcare: Current issues and recommendations for technology use. *Current Opinion in Psychology, 36*, 25–31. https://doi.org/10.1016/j.copsyc.2020.03.012

Mathews, L. (2020, April 13). *500,000 Hacked Zoom accounts given away for free on the dark web*. Forbes. https://www.forbes.com/sites/leemathews/2020/04/13/500000-hacked-zoom-accounts-given-away-for-free-on-the-dark-web/?sh=7406afc458c5

Okereafor, K., & Manny, P. (2020). Understanding cybersecurity challenges of telecommuting and video conferencing applications in the Covid-19 pandemic. *International Journal in IT & Engineering, 8*(6), 13–23. https://doi.org/10.6084/m9.figshare.12421049

Pranggono, B., & Arabo, A. (2020). COVID-19 pandemic cybersecurity issues. *Internet Technology Letters, 4*(2), Article e247. https://doi.org/10.1002/itl2.247

Ralston, W. (2020, December 9). *A dying man, a therapist and the ransom raid that shook the world*. Wired. https://www.wired.co.uk/article/finland-mental-health-data-breach-vastaamo

Ralston, W. (2021, May 4). *They told their therapists everything: Hackers leaked it all*. Wired. https://www.wired.com/story/vastaamo-psychotherapy-patients-hack-data-breach/

Zoombombing. (2021, December 3). *In Wikipedia*. https://en.wikipedia.org/wiki/Zoombombing

Chapter 5

Cyberattacks

Introduction

This chapter is the first of three looking at specific cyberthreats to practitioners. In this chapter, the focus starts with the most pertinent threats a practitioner should be aware of, involving the cyberspace and something malicious being installed on a device. The cyberattacks covered typically result in data being taken and used to extort money from the practitioner. The second chapter focuses on scams that involve the use of elements that may or may not be connected to the cyberspace (e.g. internet, email, spoofed calls). These fraud types do not typically involve infiltration of a device and often involve the victim responding to a story tailored to their profession or work as a practitioner. The third chapter focuses on payment fraud scenarios connected to day-to-day expenses you might expect to pay in your practice, where a victim can be tricked into making a payment they believe is genuine to a fraudster.

Each of these chapters provides information, action points and mitigation tips.

Later in the book, Chapter 8 on data and ethics will highlight overarching points on how only a cybersecure practice can meet professional requirements such as confidentiality, privacy and data security.

This chapter provides and enables:

Understanding

of the top threats to practitioners

Awareness

of how to spot red flags and react to them
of how to be alert and prepared to react should anything occur.

New view

of the importance of the foundations in the previous chapters
of how some of the action points and steps taken so far have created a layered defence and why these layers are important.

*

DOI: 10.4324/9781003184805-6

Overarching information

Before moving to the content of this chapter, this particular section covers some information that is pertinent to this chapter and the following two. The chapters are divided to show three groups that graduate from threats that rely on the cyberspace through to threats that rely on the victims fully falling for a deception.

Terminology

Many of the cyberattacks practitioners face lead to fraud. As per the Association of Certified Fraud Examiners [ACFE] (n.d.) fraud comprises of crimes with deception at the centre, where something is taken from another through unfair or deceptive means. It should be said that not all cybercrime is financially motivated – some perpetrators are looking to cause disruption, mischief, perform espionage or show that a company is not as protected as it should be. That said, the predominant motivating factor is monetary gain.

Another new term before continuing – "threat actor", which means the group, entity, person that might be attempting to conduct a cybercrime. It will be used in the next pages and applied interchangeably with the terms "fraudster" or "criminal", with by and large all of the terms expressing the person conducting the attack.

Reframing impact

This chapter and the next two will outline cyberthreats that can impact a practice in different ways:

Financially

- Through loss of earnings due to down-time or loss of clients due to an event
- Through an incident resulting in monetary loss or extortion (paying a ransom, fraud or theft)
- Through costs related to recovery from a data breach (fees to lawyers, rebuilding costs)

Loss of reputation

- Through a resulting data breach
- Through loss of confidential client data

This can sound a little daunting, so as you read, if anything does start to create any feeling of concern, do pause and reframe. Remember, unless you explore this material you will not be able to mitigate or respond to any of the threats. If you don't read it, you remain very firmly at risk of any of the threats, as you will never see the red flags. This material is part of taking positive steps towards protecting your practice rather than looking away and hoping it doesn't happen.

Through applying the actions in the previous chapters, many best practices will now be in operation around your client data, and you are already on a path to preventing much of what you read as best as possible. Do step into the new information in the next chapters feeling confident rather than afraid. One of the reasons these chapters step up into more detail about threats is that, at this point, you are ready to absorb this and be provided with pointers on how to react in the eventuality that something does get past the defences you have enabled.

This chapter will cover attacks where there is a predominant technological element and something is installed over the cyberspace or via a physical breach. These cyber-driven threats enable extraction of data. Cybercrimes where data can be breached lead to the opportunities for the criminal discussed earlier in this book, with data as a means to extort money, and healthcare a targeted industry due to the potential value of obtaining sensitive data. This is what happened in the Finland therapy centre case that led to dramatic press headlines (Heikkilä & Cerulus, 2020). Now you will see in this chapter how the cyberattacks behind these incidents unfold. All of the threats discussed in this chapter can impact a practice both financially and through damaging its reputation and the breach of data will need reporting to any relevant authorities and to clients.

Cyberattacks

In these pages we look at some of the cyberthreats relevant to practitioners where the two end points are online. First there is a form of installation involved. This happens either over a vulnerability or where a human enables (knowingly or unknowingly) an entry point. The result is, something unauthorised ends up on one of your devices through different possible means, such as over the internet, network or intranet. There can also be a physical breach, where something external inserted is infected (USB drive, storage drive or other) The outcome is that an external party gains unauthorised access and may be enabled to perform further actions.

Malware

The term "hacking" is commonly used today when someone illegally gains access to systems, networks, devices and accounts. Malware is one way of gaining that access. Malware can be used by a threat actor to gain access to your device or network to view or obtain your files, potentially including your banking information and credentials as well. Terms you have likely heard over time are virus, worms, trojans, adware, ransomware, along with newer or more technical terms such as rootkits, spyware, bots, fileless malware, stalkerware, keyloggers – all these fall under malware (along with others).

Consider malware as being anything that gets installed to cause harm of some kind. Malware is a common threat that impacts businesses from all industries as well as private individuals. In Chapter 1, many of the stories highlighted involved a breach of client data through malware being installed.

How it happens

Ultimately, any door you leave open into your network, device, application, software or other is one that malware can come in through. The action points in the previous chapters would have put in some layers of security to help you close many of the doors.

Importantly, in this chapter and the next ones, a new vital layer in this defence is yourself. Remember the human factor mentioned a few times. Always think before you click and respond to anything new, unexpected or changed.

The word "anything" here is important – malware can be in anything that can be transmitted. It can come in via your network or a product you use. Other examples:

Attachments or links in a forum
Attachments you download
Links or attachments added in the chat function of video conferences
Links received over email, chat or via another source
Web-browser links
Pop-ups
USB stick or storage drives
Apps, software, etc. can themselves be malware or contain malware
Add-ons (screen savers, extensions, plug-ins)

Pause for thought

No matter how curious you are, if a pop-up, link, download or USB stick/drive "appears" in your presence that you were not expecting, pause. If what you see has appeared with no explanation, do not go ahead and click on it or use it. If it is not yours – treat it that way. Never click, download or insert anything you have not expected and not verified thoroughly. If it's not something you have requested or need, don't click, activate or use it.

Why practitioners need to mitigate the risk of malware

For the practitioners reading this book, malware puts at risk all information on clients held on a device, but also essentially anything else you have stored on the device and potentially other devices on the network affected.

Those executing malware are often patient, and victims do not always notice instantly that someone behind the scenes is working out what to do with the information they have gained access to. With malware, a fraudster can gain access to, copy or remove a host of information a practitioner holds. They can then sell the data, reveal it or even destroy it on the original device. Criminals may also use it to extort money from the practitioner, or the person they sell it to may do this – more on this will be covered under ransomware, coming up next.

The extent of harm someone with unauthorised access to your device will be able to cause will depend on how good their malware is and how good your security is.

Some very complex and hard-to-detect forms of malware are now actively used that we will circle back on in the prevention section coming up. It only takes one open door or some lapses in security for a skilled criminal to cause some damage. Remember, we discussed, for example, the risk of older OSs? One security company estimates that Windows 7 is almost three times more likely to be infected than Windows 10, with an estimated 125% increase of attacks on Windows 7 in 2020 (Webroot, 2020).

All practitioners are susceptible

It can be tempting to think that only the big corporations and institutions are attacked. Larger corporations are attacked due to the money that can be elicited from them. However, smaller companies and individuals are also targeted, particularly now that the focus on home offices has increased (Marks, 2020). Verified, independent, global data on cyberattacks is difficult to find. Data often comes from security companies, which compile it in different ways they have themselves established. The statistics available still arguably provide good illumination on trends and situations. Webroot (2020) suggest that, in 2020, 62% of malware infections were related to consumer (home user) devices, compared with 38% being in business systems. The message: don't consider yourself out of the picture if you run a smaller practice or operate on your own.

What happens after malware is installed?

The following list is not exhaustive, but shows the potential results of a malware attack:

1. **Stolen credentials (usernames, passwords)**
2. **Email hacked and accessed**
3. **Files and data copied, locked and/or deleted or damaged**
4. **Financial data and bank account login credentials exposed**

5. **Computer malfunctions or acts differently or incorrectly**
6. **Further software installed now that the intruders have access to your PC**

Most cybercriminals are ultimately looking for opportunities that lead to financial gain for them. So, malware is often the key in – and after that another action will happen where they will attempt to gain from what they find. So, once in your system, the rest depends on their skills and the opportunities presented to them.

Prevention

You are operating a business that holds confidential data, so at this point, it should be clear why a good security software product was recommended earlier in the book – and particularly one providing real-time malware coverage. If you have now implemented a good product, then it will be doing its job trying to protect you from malware.

Malware is a very serious threat, and some forms are very sophisticated. So, security software that will mitigate this best are those that are regularly updated, as your security product needs to know that form of malware (have it in its database to make a match) and also be good enough to stop it. Even then, a sophisticated malware can be polymorphic and keep changing its code to stay out of sight. Note that some security products, particularly the free scanning tools mentioned earlier, may not operate on a real-time basis. They can still pick up on malware where their database has that form in it, but if they do not run real-time, it may only pick up on the malware long after it is installed (for example when you next manually run a scan).

Detection

If you find, at some point, that malware is on your computer, revert to the action points section in this chapter for initial next steps as well as those by appropriate parties in your location, such as government, law enforcement and legislative. You might need to investigate how long the malware has been on your device and gain some information about the attack before you report it. What you will need to report will depend on the data privacy and other legislation where you are situated.

One of the reasons you need to investigate what has happened is because you work with confidential data and you will need to find out if any of it has been compromised. To establish this, and remove the malware, you are strongly recommended to seek the help of a security professional who has experience in handling this kind of incident. Bear in mind that if you try to remove the malware yourself and do not fully clean your computer and other devices on the same network, not understanding what has happened (and where the exposure originated), your clients may continue to be exposed. Some malware is difficult to remove even after a full reset or re-install.

Bear in mind a malware attack can result in many outcomes, not just that your data is compromised. If you experience a malware attack, check the list provided earlier "What happens after malware is installed?" as well as the action points coming later in the chapter to help you determine what to check might have been impacted as well as your first steps in response.

*

Ransomware

Ransomware is a specific type of malware. It is prominently used today as it has proven to be very lucrative for criminals. A business may have fallen victim to it every 14 seconds in 2019 (Purplesec, n.d.). To paint a bleak but very real picture, ransomware has become a very serious global problem that is expanding:

> *Ransomware is not just financial extortion; it is a crime that transcends business, government, academic, and geographic boundaries. It has [. . .] shut down schools, hospitals, police stations, city governments, and U.S. military facilities. It is also a crime that funnels both private funds and tax dollars toward global criminal organisations. The proceeds stolen from victims may be financing illicit activities ranging from human trafficking to the development and proliferation of weapons of mass destruction.*
> *Ransomware Task Force, 2021.*

The "delay" between breaching a company and executing the data extraction, mentioned in Chapter 1, is sometimes because ransomware is often deployed after another form of malware has been installed and the threat actors have gained a foothold in your system. Once ready they deploy ransomware which will immobilise the system and operations until the victim pays a ransom demand.

➤ Data is fully locked up, encrypted or removed
➤ Victims are often threatened that their data will be exposed, sold or fully deleted if the ransom is not paid

Ransomware has been used against individuals and business owners of all sizes of business and very prominently within the healthcare sector. Many of the cases noted in Chapter 1 were of ransomware. The European Union Agency for Cybersecurity (ENISA, 2020) estimated that more than 66% of healthcare organisations experienced a ransomware attack in 2019, threat actors being all too aware of the sensitivity of the data they have access to and encouraged by the fact that many will pay a ransom to keep the data from going public or being deleted permanently. The impact of the loss of medical/health-related data does not need a lot of explaining.

Practitioners hold names and contact information of clients plus notes from sessions. Exposure of all or part of this can heavily impact a client.

Ransomware started out relatively simple: data was locked or encrypted, and you paid to get it released or get a decryption key. However, exfiltration of the data is now occurring more and more (Coveware, 2021), with cybercriminals aware that a lot of money can been made from extortion threats around selling or exposing it. In 2021, there were record cases of threat actors performing double extortion – where they both claim a ransom and still sell the data (Muhammad, 2021). Currently, there are also signs that threat actors are starting to deploy ransomware faster (Paganini, 2021), cutting down the gap in time where they gain access to a system with malware before deploying ransomware.

Ransomware is very complex to deal with. Any practitioner falling victim to it will face the dilemmas that come with this cybercrime, including the following:

- Paying up means you are paying a criminal and incurring financial loss
- Not paying means your files/data may be erased or they may be published on the darknet or elsewhere, exposing your clients
- Not all fraudsters will do as they say; some may still sell the data after a ransom is paid
- Note that regardless of the decisions made, a data breach will have to be reported since data is exposed

Variations of ransomware include the following:

- Where a ransom is not received by the deadline, some criminals might offer the victim a second chance – but for a higher fee, putting on more pressure
- Double extortion methods, as mentioned, are sometimes applied with some, or all of the exposed data being put up for sale on the darknet as well as a ransom being demanded. Or, the threat actors contact the individuals they find in the data, to extort them directly as well as extorting the company the data has been taken from
- Victims have fallen for fake "decryption tools" being marketed as genuine "solutions" purporting to decrypt files for free. Instead of doing that – once downloaded – the tools submit the victim to a second round of ransomware

If you are a practitioner who also spends time researching or working at an educational institution, you may start to note going forward news stories on ransomware attacks within both the healthcare and education sectors. In 2019, of the 72 secondary schools interviewed in a UK government survey, 76% said they had experienced a breach or an attack. For universities, the rate was around 80% for the 27 contacted. (DCMS, 2020).

You will see stories of victims paying a ransom. The decision to pay or not pay a ransom goes deep into the set-up and situated context of each case, accompanied by what would be lost or exposed. This is a complex ethical discussion for a deeper dive in another book or a future edition, as it is a topic that can expand to other dimensions.

With malware and ransomware, prevention is the only mitigation there is. Once executed, you are exposed to a potential breach scenario of anything and everything.

Further reading

Do look up ransomware and the healthcare sector if you have found some of this illuminating, as there is much to discover. Some references were placed at the end of the first chapter related to the examples discussed there. Additionally, a simple online search will find new articles.

Cyberattack first aid

Upon discovering any cyber incident, disconnect your device fully from any and all networks (Wi-Fi, internet, intranet, Bluetooth, any NFC connection or other). Whatever has infiltrated your device/network is going to still be there – disconnecting it from all possible networks may halt any remaining data from being transmitted out. It will also stop any further malware transmission across the network to other devices. Remember passive/active attacks, malware can be on a computer a while before detection and exfiltration of data has started (Coveware, 2021), perhaps your security software detected it due to an update or it starting to activate. So always go offline to protect any data that may not have left already. Until the malware is removed, do not reconnect to a network and do not use the device.

It is also recommended to fully switch off the network the device with the malware is connected to, until a qualified professional establishes the cause and extent of the infection. Do not be tempted to continue to use the network with another device until you are clear where the infection is exactly.

Action points if you experience a cyberattack

The following is aimed at the self-employed and at small businesses that do not have alternative procedures in place. They form the first basic steps to take if you become aware of a cyberattack on your practice. The list is by no means intended as an exclusive advice guide. If you have alternative procedures for your company, you should follow those, and depending on the severity of the incident, you may need to consult a cybersecurity professional.

Alternatively, or in addition, take advice from any government-level authorities where you operate, and the police, as needed. For example, the US Secret Service (n.d.) issues guides on handling cyber incidents; you can find similar resources in the country where you operate.

Steps to consider taking:

1. Stay calm; what has happened has happened. The more cool headed you are in reacting, the better

2. Disconnect the internet from your device. Also disable the Wi-Fi, Bluetooth and any data-sharing capabilities (e.g. NFC). If a phone/tablet, remove any SIM cards as well

3. Consider to call a professional. Ask the professional for any other immediate steps you should take and for their advice if they can help you find out what has happened, so you know the impact to your data, and to help you remove the malware

4. In all cases call your bank. Even if you have just noticed the cyberattack and cannot see any exposure on your bank accounts, you should always still call your bank. Financial crime does not always occur at the moment of credentials being stolen. It can happen later. Even if your accounts have not been touched yet, they might still be exposed. Your bank will advise you around securing your login credentials and cards and may be able to add you to a "watch" list. If your accounts have been exposed, your bank will direct you on the next action steps

5. From how you discovered the cyber incident and what the security professional (from point 3) finds out, you will have an idea of how severe the impact will be. You will need to change all your login credentials. When changing credentials due to a security breach, always change your security questions also, if there were any. It will feel like a large task, so keep a clear head. Write a list. Start with anything connected to client data and financial services (booking systems, email, banks, cards, shopping apps that have your cards attached). Then list all your software accounts with logins. Prioritise anything that does not have MFA too

6. If any client data on your affected device has been (or may have been) exposed and breached, you likely need to disclose and report this to the relevant authorities in your country. Refer to local data/privacy legislation (including GDPR if in EU) and guidelines, as well as your country's local data protection commissioner or equivalent for information and the steps you will need to take

7. If the cyber incident leads to financial loss, your bank will advise you where to report it. Even if there is no fraud/loss, law enforcement agencies in some countries and regions encourage all cybercrime to be reported. Check if this

is the case for your location. If you are in Europe, the Europol report a crime website is one resource for finding reporting links for different countries: https://www.europol.europa.eu/report-a-crime/report-cybercrime-online

Note that you will not always notice a cyber event immediately as it happens. It might only be later, when the attack becomes active, that you start to suspect something, or the attackers take action to block your computer (ransomware). Cybercriminals can be very patient.

Specific points regarding ransomware attacks

If you become victim to ransomware, there is a very real chance that your data will ultimately be exposed, whatever you do. Decisions to pay or not pay a ransom are complex and not something for this book to take a stance on.

The very few decryption tools out there for unlocking a ransomware-infected device (No More Ransom, n.d.) are currently rarely a solution. Those that exist are for very few of the many types of ransomware that are out there. They need to be run by a professional who has discovered precisely what you have been infected with, and then you still need to be lucky that there is a tool for that exact version. Decryption tools do not solve that the threat actor may have already gained access to your data. They purely might help unlock it. This means, for practitioners they offer little value except potential access to your data if you have no other backup.

After a ransomware attack, whether a ransom is paid or not, impacted devices (and in some cases networks) need to be fully sanitised and enhanced security added to prevent the same attack again. Where the ransom is not paid, if you have a backup of files offline, you can reload them after the impacted devices have been sanitised and restarted. We will look more at the topic of backup files in Chapter 8.

There is a brief checklist at the back of the book with some tips on recovery after a cyberattack.

Let's take a break from learning about cyberattacks to reflect on two case studies, around topics written about in the book so far.

Sandra's case – Part 1

Sandra decides to finally buy a handbag she has been thinking about getting; it is a bit expensive but there are sales online right now, and she recently found out that she is due for a refund from the government for lost earnings due to her practice being forced to close for some months. She had replied to their email last week with the information they had asked for, including her lost earnings in good time, and had provided the rest of the banking information they needed when they called this week, so that will come in soon. After a quick look for the cheapest merchant, she selects the bag, clicks to check out and adds in her name, address and credit card info. After clicking place order, up comes the final screen for her to enter her MFA code. Without hesitating, Sandra adds the code and clicks confirm.

Payment denied.

Sandra tries again but faces the same problem. She knows she has enough in her account, so she is a little confused. She opens a new screen and logs in to check her bank account. A couple of hard looks at the screen leave her wondering if she needs new glasses.

All her accounts and her credit card have a minus next to them.

Knowing the first thing to do is call the bank, she does so, explaining that there has been a big mistake!

Activity

Open your reflective notes and start a page called "Sandra".

What do you think has happened to Sandra?
Would you have done anything differently purchasing the bag?
What else might you do as well as call the bank?

Case study break – Perky

Now is a good time to read another full case study before reading on. Turn to the back of the book and look up "The Full Case of Perky" (p. 171). These studies build on some of the knowledge so far and will enable you to practise your reaction to the information given in the case study as the story builds.

Try not to be tempted to read the final Level 3 case study afterwards. Wait until it comes up in the book. Re-reading the Level 1 study is fine though. You might note through doing so whether you are starting to spot and absorb the information in new ways. Each of the case studies is set up to give you opportunities to tune your cyberthreat radar and either covers territory you have crossed or territory coming up soon.

Take your time with them, as the reflective element will help you see how you are moving your learning into your own application of it.

*

Institution and corporate-level view

For practitioners who are also the following:

- Researchers or educators at educational establishments
- Contracted to or employed by corporates
- Employed as associates
- Volunteers for charities

The threats covered so far illuminate why many companies will ask you to undergo training in cybersecurity or another security-related domain. Many companies and institutions will also have expectations from you when it comes to data storage. By now you have seen that this is a world where criminals will reach for the data they can see and take for themselves. Understanding your role in helping a corporation or institution keep data safe is vital.

1. Larger institutions, corporations and companies will have cybersecurity teams. They will be combating threats on a daily basis. Therefore, they have reasons for the cyber policies, procedures and training they implement
2. An institution, corporation or company may ask you to use one tool over another. For example, a particular video conferencing tool or specific cloud storage tool. The decision to use these products may come from cyber incidents in the past, regulations that are imposed on them from overarching authorities/bodies or simply that they are narrowing down to specific tools they believe are safer to use than others. If you have questions about the tools and why they've been chosen, ask them; however, do use the tools they state in policies and procedures unless you gain permission to do otherwise
3. Remember, a corporation you work for may be a very different business compared with your profession. For example, you may be coaching in a manufacturing company. Manufacturing companies, too, are regularly targeted for their data (Lemos, 2021) – on what they make, build or create. The knowledge you have built of cybercrime for your profession and practice will help you understand how others can be targeted and why you might be restricted in the tools you can use when working for them
4. Embrace the friction when you are required to use a tool you are not acquainted with over one you know or would have preferred. See it as a learning experience and remember the reason you are asked to use that product might be to keep your participants' data (and your research data) as well as the company/institution safe and secure
5. A topic for expansion in another edition is that practitioners who are working in the education sector can be part of helping drive the change in cyber awareness with students of psychology, coaching, counselling and therapy. When writing up experiences working with test clients, the cyber risks that come with sharing data with an institution need to be known thoroughly by the participants. Students also

need to be protected from responsibility in the event of a data breach on a university system – of their assignments, which often contain confidential material from conversations with test clients (e.g. Moodle has been extensively hacked: Rashid, 2021). Information is available (NCSC, 2021); it just needs to be much better applied. This topic will need to be explored more in the near future

*

Cyber liability insurance

This is noted here primarily so that you know it exists, if you did not already. Whether this is something for your practice is up to each reader. If you already have some form of business insurance, one option is investigating whether cyber liability insurance can be added to your existing coverage.

What does it cover?

It depends on the insurance provider and the policy taken, but it can cover aspects such as recovery costs incurred as a result of a cyber incident, advice on what to do, support reporting the incident. It might also cover costs of any legal action around a data breach from underlying individuals, clients or authorities. Check carefully the details of what each provider you consider might cover.

Important considerations

An insurance policy will often come with expectations on how you have secured your practice, to start with. If you do take out cyber liability insurance, ensure to read the terms and conditions carefully and ensure you can meet them.

It is difficult to provide data to say how much a cyber incident, or breach, costs a company or victim. Widely different data is available, and much is at country level (Hiscox Limited, 2020). Additionally, cyber insurance will likely either become more expensive over time or need to change in structure. This is due to the challenge it has to balance premiums versus the at·times very heavy payouts to clients (Johansmeyer, 2021). Also, while some cyber insurers issue policies that include reimbursing ransoms paid out to criminals, some are now no longer doing this (Bajak, 2021). Paying ransoms has not been free of controversy (Barbaschow, 2020). Where governments and authorities may condemn it today, worth knowing is that many of them have, in the past, turned a blind eye and even paid ransoms themselves (Deloitte, 2020) . This is a deeply difficult problem to resolve as threat actors are not just after data they can sell; some are creating national threats by infiltrating, for example, governments, the military and nuclear facilities (Sharma, 2021; Ransomware Task Force, 2021). Put simply, there is data in the world that once lost or placed in the wrong hands could cause irreparable damage.

Summary

The chapter has covered the top threats practitioners may face that rely on use of the cyberspace to execute. These threats are also some of the most used, and most lucrative for cybercriminals. Monetary loss from global cybercrime was estimated by one cybersecurity company as totalling US\$ 945 billion by 2020, or 1% of the world's GDP (Malekos & Lostri, 2020). The IT-Security Institute AV Test, at the time of writing this, registered over 350,000 new malicious programs daily, and recorded a total malware count for the end of 2021 of 1312.64m programs (AV Test, 2022). ENISA (2020) estimated that €10.1 billion in ransoms were paid in 2019, with 45% of companies paying up in the event of a ransom attack, and only half of those actually getting their data back.

It was estimated that, in 2021, there were 3.5 million unfilled cybersecurity jobs (Morgan, 2021). As covered earlier, you may be your own cybersecurity. Through explaining the top cyberthreats faced by a practitioner, this chapter has enabled the following resources to your cybersecurity toolkit:

- Ability now to more easily absorb articles in the media about cyber incidents. Previously, the terminology may have seemed complex, or the topic alarming. Now, the practitioner is aware of much of the basics
- Clarity and background to why you have been putting in some good foundational defences via the previous chapters
- A basic understanding of some starter action points if a cyber incident occurs

An important part of any cybersecurity setup is the human factor (Back & LaPrade, 2019). Therefore, the next chapters (6 and 7), focus on how to spot scams and fraud attempts aimed at practitioners.

References

Association of Certified Fraud Examiners. (n.d.). *What is fraud?* https://www.acfe.com /fraud-101.aspx

AV Test. (2022). *Malware.* https://www.av-test.org/en/statistics/malware/

Back, S., & LaPrade, J. (2019). The future of cybercrime prevention strategies: Human factors and a holistic approach to cyber intelligence. *International Journal of Cybersecurity Intelligence & Cybercrime, 2*(2), 1–4. https://www.doi.org/10.52306/02020119KDHZ8339

Bajak, F. (2021, May 9). Insurer AXA to stop paying for ransomware crime payments in France. *Insurance Journal.* https://www.insurancejournal.com/news/international/2021/ 05/09/613255.htm

Barbaschow, A. (2020, August 4). *Cyber insurance: The moral quandary of paying criminals who stole your data.* ZDNet. https://www.zdnet.com/article/cyber-insurance-the-moral-quandary-of-paying-criminals-who-stole-your-data/

Coveware. (2021, February 1). *Ransomware payments fall as fewer companies pay data exfiltration extortion demands.* https://www.coveware.com/blog/ransomware-marketplace-report-q4-2020

Deloitte Center for Government Insights. (2020). *Ransoming government: What state and local governments can do to break free from ransomware attacks.* Deloitte Insights. https://www2.deloitte.com/content/dam/insights/us/articles/6421_Ransoming-government/DI_Ransoming-government.pdf

Department for Digital, Culture, Media and Sport (DCMS). (2020). *Cyber security breaches survey 2020: Education institutions findings annex.* Gov.UK. Crown Copyright. https:// www.gov.uk/government/statistics/cyber-security-breaches-survey-2020

Europol. (n.d.). *Report cybercrime online.* https://www.europol.europa.eu/report-a-crime/report-cybercrime-online

The European Union Agency for Cybersecurity (ENISA). (2020). *ENISA threat landscape 2020 – ransomware.* https://www.enisa.europa.eu/publications/ransomware

Heikkilä, M., & Cerulus, L. (2020, October 26). Hacker seeks to extort Finnish mental health patients after data breach. *Politico.* https://www.politico.eu/article/cybercriminal-extorts-finnish-therapy-patients-in-shocking-attack-ransomware-blackmail-vastaamo/

Hiscox Limited. (2020). *The Hiscox cyber readiness report 2020.* https://www.hiscoxgroup.com/sites/group/files/documents/2020-06/Hiscox-Cyber-Readiness-Report-2020.pdf

Johansmeyer, T. (2021, January 11). *Cybersecurity insurance has a big problem.* Harvard Business Review. https://hbr.org/2021/01/cybersecurity-insurance-has-a-big-problem

Lemos, R. (2021, June 18). *One in five manufacturing firms targeted by cyberattacks.* Dark Reading. https://beta.darkreading.com/attacks-breaches/one-in-five-manufacturing-firms-targeted-by-cyberattacks

Malekos, Z., & Lostri, E. (2020). *The hidden costs of cybercrime.* McAfee. https://www.mcafee.com/enterprise/en-us/assets/reports/rp-hidden-costs-of-cybercrime.pdf

Marks, G. (2020, July 16). Here's another virus terrorising businesses and causing havoc: Ransomware. *The Guardian.* https://www.theguardian.com/business/2020/jul/16/small-business-malware-ransomware-working-from-home

Morgan, S. (2021, November 9). *Cybersecurity jobs report: 3.5 million openings in 2025.* Cyber Security Ventures. https://cybersecurityventures.com/jobs/

Muhammad, Z. (2021, December 17). *2021 saw record breaking number of double extortion ransomware attacks.* Digital Information World. https://www.digitalinformationworld.com/2021/12/2021-saw-record-breaking-number-of.html

National Cyber Security Centre. (2021, June 4). *Alert: Further ransomware attacks on the UK education sector by cyber criminal.* Crown Copyright. https://www.ncsc.gov.uk/news/alert-targeted-ransomware-attacks-on-uk-education-sector

No More Ransom. (n.d.). https://www.nomoreransom.org/en/index.htm

Paganini, P. (2021, December 8). *Emotet directly drops Cobalt Strike beacons without intermediate Trojans.* Security Affairs. https://securityaffairs.co/wordpress/125384/cyber-crime/emotet-cobalt-strike.html

Purplesec. (n.d.). *The growing threat of ransomware.* https://purplesec.us/resources/cyber-security-statistics/ransomware/

Ransomware Task Force. (2021). Prepared by the institute for security and technology. *Combatting Ransomware.* https://securityandtechnology.org/wp-content/uploads/2021/04/IST-Ransomware-Task-Force-Report.pdf

Rashid, H. (2021, April 12). *6-year-old Moodle flaw exposed millions to account takeover attack.* HackRead. https://www.hackread.com/6-year-old-moodle-account-takeover-vulnerability/

Sharma, M. (2021, June 15). *US nuclear weapons supplier hit by ransomware attack.* TechRadar. https://www.techradar.com/news/us-nuclear-weapons-supplier-hit-by-ransomware-attack

United States Secret Service. (n.d.). *Preparing for a cyber incident.* https://www.secretservice.gov/investigation/Preparing-for-a-Cyber-Incident

Webroot. (2020). *Webroot threat report.* https://mypage.webroot.com/rs/557-FSI-195/images/2020%20Webroot%20Threat%20Report_US_FINAL.pdf

Chapter 6

Scams tailored to your profession

Introduction

In this chapter, we will cover some of the scams and fraud scenarios tailored to the professions of the readers of this book. In all the cases covered, the scam relies on you partnering with the fraudster to execute. The word "partnering" is used here to illuminate that the victim does take part in some way, by responding to a hook. This hook may be an emotional story, an incredible offer or a solution to a problem. Later, the victim may look back at the situation and wonder why they fell for the story or question their actions. At the time, however, they may have been unaware of what was happening, may not have seen the red flags, may have been pressured into a decision or felt they didn't have another option. The word "complicit" is avoided and not used as fraudsters manipulate and coerce in ways that can lure anyone in where they find the right time and the right story when talking to their victims.

Many of the threats that are covered next you can prevent by spotting the red flags before you end up being pulled into participating. That is, developing just a little extra awareness on how these fraud attempts are executed and learning to respond to red flags and abnormal behaviour, can help practitioners avoid the fallout from financial crime, noted earlier, which includes the following:

- Disruption of business
- Financial loss
- Damage to reputation

Beyond your practice

The focus is on the attacks most likely to occur in relation to the professional practice areas of the audience of this book. However, most of the scams and phishing attempts that will be shown actually use similar underlying elements, methods and MO when used on other populations. So, as well as keeping clients safer, an added incentive: the underlying knowledge will improve your radar to spotting where you are being manipulated, giving you improved defences throughout all areas of your cyber life.

DOI: 10.4324/9781003184805-7

A number of fraud scenarios that have been experienced by practitioners are presented. Some of these could occur with other small businesses in other industries. As will be shown, criminals often create a theme or story around what they are doing, so that it fits the reality of a particular business. From seeing the way the stories are applied, and the underlying cybercrime, you can build a skill set we have been starting to construct already through the case studies so far – aimed at enhancing your ability to see red flags and react to them.

Even with crimes that focus on eliciting money from you, bear in mind that these can also impact reputation – since any kind of cyber-enabled incident indicates a lack of security in an environment holding trusted information. This chapter and book does not cover all possible scams that can be aimed at you, and all the ways to stop them. It aims to help build your competences to help you stop what you can. Do continue to read any and all alerts sent to you by authorities, banks and other sources on an ongoing basis.

Outcomes from this chapter include the following:

Protective foundations

Through knowledge of some of the ways to detect and mitigate the threats described

Understanding of how individuals become vulnerable

Through noting how fraudsters aim to emotionally manipulate their potential victims

Ability to react

Confidence to know how to react, the first steps and where to look to proceed

*

Scams tailored to your profession

Before tackling some of the scams that have been targeted specifically towards your professions, a refresh of some terminology you may have some knowledge of from alerts in the media or from banks and authorities.

Scams

Scams are aimed at exploiting money. For a practitioner, this may therefore not always lead to data loss or a data breach. Many codes of ethics require that the practitioner positively represent their profession, however, and there can be a ripple effect from being a victim of fraud – one that can impact a business practice with financial loss, disruption to business and, potentially, loss of reputation.

There can also always be an emotional and mental health impact with all types of fraud on victims, with many experiencing problems in the aftermath (Button et al., 2014). Not becoming a victim to cases such as those in this chapter will keep the practitioner running a healthy practice that can serve its clients.

Scammers tell a story to lure you into making a decision to provide money. Due to extensive media coverage and life experience, many reading this will be able to cite a number of scams.

Some scams are done through adverts, emails or online. Examples include the investments offered on a popular social media site that sound too good to be true and the lure of an email that comes at a time when you are looking for precisely what it is offering. The difference compared with the ransomware and malware attacks noted earlier is that most type of scams require social engineering or manipulation of people rather than installation of something into your technology.

Phishing

Phishing is essentially a specific method a threat actor uses to uncover sensitive information from a victim for their own gain. Phishing is traditionally associated with emails, but due to the expansion of techniques, other terms – such as smishing (over SMS), vhishing (over calls) and spear phishing (where the contact is directed specifically at a person) – have come up. It can also involve spoofing – spoofed websites, email senders, telephone numbers as part of the attack. In the rest of the book, phishing is used in a collective sense to cover all these variations.

Peeling off the labels and terms, it may be easier to understand that phishing leads to sensitive information being revealed – either by the victims themselves providing it in response to something or through malware being installed by a victim clicking something and enabling unauthorised access to their device.

Social engineering

Your profession is a setting or environment that can be leveraged in a scam story. Through that the scammer has access to you, and from there to financial gain – by manipulating the weakest links. Operating as a practitioner, you may have information about yourself online. Scams targeting businesses can cover a wide range – think of Mark from earlier. This was essentially a tax scam involving vhishing, spoofing and social engineering. The caller used the story around tax to obtain credit card information. The tax authority number was spoofed. It could have been another story, but for the same outcome, and this is where social engineering comes in. Mark was targeted at a time of the year when small businesses were completing taxes, and his discourse revealed to the fraudster that he was not fully on top of his accounts. This became an opportunity to engineer Mark into giving up his credit card information by helping him feel supported and giving him a solution.

One way to see the emotional layer that comes up here is to consider some of the scams that happened during the COVID-19 pandemic, where many were concerned about topics such as health, wellness and infection in a heightened way.

People's vulnerability increased through fear, and they became more prone to clicking on links related to topics they were concerned about without seeing red flags. People signed up for offers that, at another time, they would have noticed were simply too good to be true, such as free shopping at a well-known supermarket (Furnell & Shah, 2020).

Pulling it together

Now that we have covered three well-used terms, let's put them in another context that shows them as elements:

Scam: this can be seen as the overarching "what" – the story presented to you – which is delivered either directly (1:1 contact, link, targeted correspondence) or indirectly (advertising, website, random pop-up, correspondence sent out en-masse)

Phishing: this is the specific method behind how you are approached to reveal sensitive information, luring you into respond with information yourself or to click on something that enables malware into your device

Social engineering: this is, in some ways, the broader packaging of how you are personally manipulated and convinced into seeing something the way the fraudster would like you to see it, rather than what it really is. Later the victim opens the beautiful packaging to find themselves disappointed or devastated by the contents

So, filtered down to bare bones, this involves the following:

- Story
- Method
- Packaging

Before moving on to look at examples of scams targeted at practitioners, a short break to look at Part 2 of Sandra's case.

Sandra's case – Part 2

In your notes after reading Part 1 (p. 105), you might have written down a number of thoughts as to what happened to Sandra. It is an option that the website she has landed on, entered information into and made a purchase from is fraudulent and harvesting payment data for further exploitation. She had looked for the cheapest way to purchase the bag and did not check the reputation of the site she used. A good price can lure people into purchasing without hesitation from a site or even a vendor on a reputable site without checking who they are buying from.

Whether purchasing for yourself or your business, always buy from a reputable online store, or a vendor with a proven track record or good reviews. Something being offered at a price that is too good to be true can be a red flag that it might either be a fake item or a non-reputable service. Often doing an internet search of the firm can help. Is there any information out there? Search the merchant's name plus "scam" and see what comes up. If you thought of this – or anything similar – as potentially explaining what happened to Sandra, congratulations. It demonstrates you are starting to think critically and look for red flags when operating online.

In Sandra's case, however, as some of you may have picked up, the timing of buying the bag does not fit with the withdrawals having *already* happened on her account. Instead, the rest of the story provides the answer. Note some subtle similarities with Mark's tax case.

Some new information

Sandra has responded to correspondence about a refund from the government in relation to her practice having to close for a period in 2020. The request had felt slightly strange as she had asked in 2020 if she was eligible for something and had been told no. However, she pushed this strange feeling away, excited about getting some money she had not expected. She quickly read through the information and responded via email, as requested, with an estimate of her lost earnings, her bank details and login information.

The email Sandra received was well constructed but from a gov1.com mail domain. Sandra was not aware that the "1" might be irregular in an email from an authority and overlooked that the UK government uses a gov.uk domain. Similarly, the information she was sent included a link to a well-constructed, replicated page of the government website, logo and all. Sandra didn't notice there were formatting issues on the gov1.com page. She could also have considered that the government had never asked her for information via email before – for anything. Finally, she missed another clue the day after she replied when they phoned her, explaining they were processing everything and just needed her to confirm some final confirmations (codes) that would arrive by SMS on her phone.

The spoofed email and website are arguably difficult to spot. There were, however, red flags from start to end that could have been noticed with the emotional layer and story peeled back.

Activity

Before reading the last paragraph of this case, read through again and write down in your reflective notes any other red flags you can see in Sandra's story.

Once you are finished with your notes, continue.

Sandra's case – Part 2 Continued

Final information

Sandra had not considered verifying why there was a change that she now was due for some support money, when the last time she had been told no. Sandra also didn't notice the nice gentleman on the phone asking for some final confirmation codes was actually asking for her for banking transaction MFA codes. She didn't read the SMS messages carefully, just gave the numbers and she did not consider the warnings she had heard before about never giving credentials to another. Essentially, she had first given her banking information to fraudsters in writing and now was giving them the final pieces so that they could log in and transfer money out. Either swept away at the thought of getting money back or convinced that the caller was from the government, Sandra did not question that a person in authority would ask her for such information. Sandra essentially participated by giving the criminal everything they needed to complete the crime.

Targeted scams

The threats in the last chapter rely on technology and the cyberspace, while in the examples coming up, technology plays a smaller part in the background and in the delivery of the scam.

While malware and data loss can still end up in an outcome of scams (and we will cover this combination at the end of this section), first described are the targeted scams where the fraudster socially engineers their victim into responding with information or an action that leads to monetary gain for the fraudster.

Unpacked are particular scams targeted at practitioners that have been disclosed. Many of the scams listed have been reported on professional body websites, such as those of the International Coaching Federation (ICF), American Psychological Association (APA) and British Association for Counselling and Psychotherapy (BACP), and other places such as private blogs. The examples are not exclusive but have been picked out as common examples where the underlying elements can be unpacked to guide you through building awareness towards spotting other (or new) scams.

Court scam/warrant scams

Note as you read, how the fraudsters involved in this try to use manipulation to arouse emotions in the practitioner, such as making them feel they have done something against the law or in violation of a code of conduct.

In this scam, the fraudster calls practitioners saying they have missed going to court in response to a subpoena to be an expert witness. This scam plays on the fact that many practitioners follow ethical guidelines that require them to hold records for a certain period of time and that can require them to appear in court as requested by authorities.

Example scenario: practitioner receives a call informing them that they have not shown up and that this has consequences. They quickly find themself in a fear-based emotional state. In this heightened state, they may overlook red flags and want to resolve this immediately. In these targeted scams, practitioners are often informed that they are at risk of arrest or criminal charges, and in some cases, that they are now being monitored (Borders, 2019; Warren-Hicks, 2020)

Once frightened or in a fear-based state, the practitioner is offered an opportunity to resolve by arranging to pay a bail bond or other arrangement in cash, such as clearing a fine. Some of the scam calls have realistic background noise (police radio), and the fraudster uses officer names that match with those in the victim's local police department as well as a spoofed police department number (Cavazos, 2018).

Activity

Open your reflective notes and add your reflections to the below points before proceeding to the next paragraph.

- Note the potential red flags you can see in the aforementioned scam
- Reflect on what you would have done if you had received this phone call
- What else comes up for you?

Each of the scenarios in this section will have a reflective section. Do take time to do the reflective exercises as they will help you to build your own responses and skills.

Once you have finished your notes, continue reading.

How to avoid being caught up in a scam like this?

Despite that you may consider yourself well educated and someone who would spot a fake story and despite some red flags and unrealistic elements in the warrant/court scam stories, some still fall for them (Cavazos, 2018; Borders, 2019; Warren-Hicks, 2020) and the other scams explored in this section – or they wouldn't be here!

The underlying elements of this scam are used against different targets. For example, teachers have been targeted via calls made to their school office claiming they have missed a court date (Wade, 2018). Private individuals are contacted and told they have missed jury service (United States Courts, n.d.).

These are examples of red flags in this scam:

- You have no recollection of having received an invitation to the court
- The person on the phone is pushy. They try to incite an emotional response in you, rather than calmly informing you about the situation
- The conversation comes with a threat (arrest or other) that needs money to resolve it. Unpacked: a negative emotional response is invoked where the "fix" is payment
- The suggestions on how to "resolve" the situation appear abnormal – irregular payment form, time pressure, irregular meeting point

How to avoid being caught up in any scam?

No matter how afraid you may feel from a story unfolded by a person talking to you or writing to you, if there is something not quite right, pause. In any and all cases of an unusual or unexpected call from somewhere, you can always request time to look into it. Take time to do the following:

- Evaluate any red flags and abnormalities
- Remember that scams come with packaging that might be tailored precisely to your taste and needs, making it harder to see the red flags. Example: you are offered something you always wanted (CPH & Associates, n.d.)
- Say you will call back, and then end the call – no matter how hard the person contacting you pushes
- Remember spoofing and social engineering – look up an official, trusted number for where the caller claimed they are from and call back using only the verified number to double-check the story
- Research and verify whether, if you have failed to do something as claimed by the person contacting you, that it would have the consequences they say it does

These points may seem very clear; yet people still fall for scams. Consider some of the case studies covered in this book so far and how the scenarios can fit into the aforementioned. Even for claims of unpaid bills, services, subscriptions – though very different in nature – if it doesn't sound right, pause to double-check thoroughly and review whether what you are being informed about is genuine.

Pre-payment scams and advanced fee scams

These are a good example of the tailoring done with scams towards practitioners' professions. By now most of the audience of this book will have had a variant or two of the original version of these scams in their spam mail folder. Claims you have won something for free or promises of a significant amount of money in return for some help moving money out of a country, the latter often with an emotional story of the money being previously trapped, taken, stolen or other and at risk of being lost unless someone can help them. These are pre-payment or advanced fee scams that unfold through the victim being engineered into having to pay postage to receive what they have won or covering the fees/cost of sending the money out of a country in advance. In other variations, victims are sent cheques and while that is clearing at the bank, they have already wired to the fraudster the equivalent money back only to find the cheque later bounces.

A version of this scam and packaging wrapped up for practitioners is that a fraudster places a call to book appointments – often for someone they know – and states that they want to pay on their behalf. They offer to pay upfront via cheque. After the practitioner receives and deposits the cheque, the fraudster places a call to say they are cancelling the appointments. They are happy for a cancellation fee to be taken but would appreciate having their money returned (Caldwell, 2009, Borders, 2021). The fraudster will request a return of funds quickly or via an instant payment system, which will mean that the victim may send the returned amount before the cheque is found out as fraudulent at the bank.

Activity

Open up your reflective notes.

- Cheques are used less and less today so think about the story and the packaging and how the underlying technique could be used in another way
- Reflect on what you would have done if you were the practitioner in this case. Would you have seen red flags? If so, what would you have done?

How to avoid this type of scam?

These are examples of red flags in this scam:

Being asked for a refund soon after a payment is made from someone you have not yet worked with

Payment being sent by someone you have not connected to thoroughly

The story of why money has been paid up front is likely emotive (helping a friend, relative)

Regarding cheques being outdated in some countries, this is true, so keep in mind the underpinning of the scam: money is claimed as sent to you at the same time you are asked to send it back. So, take care with any "proof of payment" a client produces showing money sent electronically. Always wait for any incoming money to clear on your account before you send anything back. If in doubt, talk to your bank.

Examples of adjusted versions of this scam:

* A new client claims they have paid "too much" and need a partial refund – be very alert (British Association for Counselling & Psychotherapy, [BACP], n.d.). Do some extra checks on the client and make sure the money (however it was sent; cheque or electronically) has cleared on your account before you return a partial or full amount
* Wider variations of this scam include something a practitioner has put for sale (goods for sale/rental space). The MO follows a similar pattern – cheque/payment being provided, then a change of mind and request for refund (Caldwell, 2019)

Many practitioners do not take payment before sessions, but if you do – or you take deposits for packages ahead of time – consider your procedures around this with brand new clients ahead of working with them and getting to know them.

Consider the role of social engineering in this scam. The story will often be heartfelt, an example: someone wanting to get counselling to help them through a difficult time. The trick, then, is to spot a scam behind such a story when you are in a profession of precisely wanting to provide services to help others. That's where the red flags come in. Scammers may pick their stories carefully, but they do make mistakes, and there can be something in the rest of the story that stands out as not sitting quite right.

Fake certification/training

These scams include fake offers for training, certification or other in association with an apparent school, association or body connected to your profession (Pickup, 2020).

Activity

Open up your reflective notes.

> Consider briefly: how have you verified courses you have signed up for in the past?
> What will you do going forward?
> Finish your notes before continuing.

Tips towards not being scammed by a fake course, certification or programme

- Make sure to always verify any new online school or CPD body you have not studied with before

    - Have any of your peers attended a course there?
    - Who is recommending it?
    - Do not pay anything until you have verified everything thoroughly

- Verify any accreditation or qualification claims back to the relevant professional body. Particularly if the course is run by a school you do not know, and it claims to have a fast-track or appears to have a simplified process to become accredited, licenced or other (Caldwell, 2009)
- Check out if the course is listed as CPD by the applicable CPD standards office

Other potential red flags

- Is the course promising employment or money or some kind of guarantee after?
- Read the fine print: are follow-up courses or further payments required to gain the qualification advertised in the marketing materials (Gausden, 2020)?

You can also apply elements of these red flags when evaluating offers for marketing, publicity and other support offered as services to your practice. Check if you know someone who has used the service, review thoroughly any new company and what they are offering. Don't rely only on what the advertising company sends; cross-check with other sources. Note also that with these scams the emotional response is not fear but perhaps excitement or a sense of getting something you really want/need for a good price. Any time you have the feeling that you are getting something above and beyond expectations, the "too good to be true" red flag should wave; when it does, take it as a reminder to pause and double-check everything.

Breach of practice scams

A variation of the first scam noted earlier (court scams) has involved practitioners receiving a call or contact from someone claiming to be from a government authority. The practitioner is informed that they are being prosecuted for an offence and are given a chance to pay a fine instead or lose their licence (APA Services, 2019). Here again, even where the victim has no history of anything related to what they are told, they are socially engineered into a place of fear, where some succumb to the threat and pay.

In countries where you are licenced to perform your profession – or linked to a government or other body where you are adhering to strict regulations – always be thoroughly aware of the relevant rules, regulations and framework of those bodies. This will help protect you from such scams by being aware of abnormalities in fraudsters' stories of how you have breached your licence or regulations. If you are not licenced, be aware that variations of this scam may encompass being told you've breached data legislation, ethics, other aspects relevant to your practice.

Activity

Open up your reflective notes.

Reflect on this and write some notes on what can protect you from this type of scam, before you continue.

How to avoid being caught up in this type of scam?

First – always peel back the emotional layer of what is being presented. What is it you are being informed you have breached? Does this story ring true in any way?

Make a call back to the body/authority claiming to be contacting you and verify the story with them directly (using always an official number you find and not the one given to you by the person contacting you). If you have an online account with them, you can also log in and check if anything is logged there and check the regulations.

If you have received contact by email, check the email address thoroughly. Have you received emails from them before? Keep in mind many authorities do not use regular email for correspondence, often instead requiring you to log into an account/secure service to read written correspondence. Getting an email for the first time or unexpectedly from anywhere is worth pausing to think about.

If you receive suspicious contact by post with a contact number to call, to discuss that you missed a court appearance (or other) that you were not aware of, again, look for an official main telephone number yourself and do not use the one on the letter.

Remember also that if you have genuinely missed something, an authority will confirm and be able to discuss with you resolution of this rationally and without threats.

If you are licenced by a particular board or authority, it will usually be the case that only that issuing authority can revoke the licence or certification and/or initiate disciplinary proceedings (APA Services, 2019). That is, if you are being contacted by someone claiming to be connected to a governmental department, or another party that is not the authority issuing the licence or award, this may be a red flag.

Keeping calm and a clear head helps keep control of the emotional layer; then, the abnormal elements of a scam will become more visible. You will be in a better place to recognise that one phone call and an immediate payment would unlikely be the actual solution to any real disciplinary action by an official body a practitioner is licenced or certified with. There often would be a period of investigation that the practitioner is informed about, and the first contact would likely not be one involving an immediate resolution or fee involving money. Remember the caller will be listening for when a victim is frightened enough that they might make a payment.

If the person contacting you has information about you, such as membership numbers, do not take this as proof that they are who they say they are. Information about you, your practice, numbers of your licence or other detail might have been found online. Do not take this at face-value, as indicating they are genuine callers (APA Services, 2019).

The emotional factor

One extremely important point to note is the emotional element and packaging of the scam. This is where *any* scam can catch someone out to the point that all red flags seem to disappear. Here is an example:

A variation of the court house scam, involving missed jury service, was mentioned earlier. This version of the scam is typically targeted at any individual, as jury service is something anyone can be invited to and not connected to your profession. In one account of this scam, a counsellor was informed she had missed jury duty and threatened with arrest. She became afraid her clients would hear she was arrested. Knowing this would affect her business, any and all red flags did not register. It was only after she had bought and relayed a number of gift card numbers, per the fraudster's demands, that she started to become suspicious. By then it was too late, and most of the money was lost (Cavazos, 2018).

Because practitioners are working with sensitive data and in a trusted position, some threats will automatically raise a sense of fear or nervousness without needing a lot of packaging. This example demonstrates that how we are situated, at the moment a scam is put to us, plays a role in whether we will spot it. This is why this section has unpacked elements to demonstrate the importance of always being alert to red flags and abnormalities in any story put to you.

Advertising scams

In these, a practitioner is called and asked if they would like to have an advertisement placed in a particular directory (International Coaching Federation [ICF], 2020). The caller then elicits payment up-front from the victim.

Activity

Reflect briefly on how you react to someone offering advertising, support or services. How will you verify this next time before you respond?

Tips towards not falling for these scams

Be aware how visible you may be online or in the public due to your profession. This means that someone contacting you may have quite some detail on you and be able to weave a good story about advertising that would support your practice. The more public you make your information, the more vigilant you should be with requests, as scams will come. Always verify anything you are tempted to sign up for thoroughly before making any payment.

Media, publishing and marketing scams

Where you are used to writing chapters in books, appearing on radio, helping with courses, conferences or other, you might not think about verifying a caller enquiring if you are interested in a writing proposal or a media appearance. However, the ICF (Mitten, 2017) and others have alerted on scams related to radio, books, coaching franchises and fake Google services.

How to avoid being lured by these scams?

If you are being contacted by a party you have not worked with before, pause and do some due diligence. If enticed into something you have always wanted to do, you may not see red flags such as being asked to pay towards your appearance, publication or other (Mitten, 2017) – with what you pay for, of course, never materialising.

Where you have a prominent position, title or role within your industry, fraudsters will have even more information on you available to them and will likely target you more frequently. Moreover, if you run a business as well, this puts you at play for other forms of fraud, such as CEO Fraud, which has been attempted against practitioners. We will touch upon this in Chapter 7.

Phishing and malware

This chapter has focused more on the scams that rely on a human factor, but as promised in the opening part of this section, before we close, a brief note to show where the previous chapter and this one connect. Malware, per the last chapter, is how criminals can install software that enables them unauthorised access to your data and an ability to extract that data. Phishing is one way that malware can be installed. Now that you have read various scams, it is probably easier to see how a convincing story might entice someone into clicking on something or providing access to someone that they might not do in another circumstance. In the phishing scams linked to malware, there will be at some point something to click, download, open – that will then install the malicious software on your device. Thereafter, the information in the last chapter comes into play and you can expect a data breach or further issues to come up.

In the next section, we move on to more tips on spotting red flags and being alert to abnormalities at all times.

Scams and spotting red flags

Here a little more detail is covered, using an example from the last section, on how to unpack a story in a way that may reveal a scam.

Fraudsters will use their knowledge of your professional work as psychologists, therapists, coaches, counsellors to target particular emotional points. They are aware you are trained to practice high ethical standards and work in professions wanting to help people. Manipulating a practitioner into believing something, and/or of being afraid, means that they are more likely to fall victim to a story.

Being alert

Break down the elements of any story being told to you.

Separate yourself from the emotional layers as you dig into what is going on and unpack the story being told.

What is it that is actually being presented?

What is being stated?

Is it feasible?

An example using the court case scam

Story and emotional layer

Story: you failed to turn up to a court case
Emotional layer: severe consequences

Potential fear response

Fear of not being able to operate as a practitioner
Sense of failure to do due duty
Fear of damage to your reputation
Impact of consequences

New response

Remove the emotion and unpack the story and the view looks different.
Story: you know you can be called to court, but you do not recall a request.

Emotional layer: the consequences are understandable, but arrest and a fine will need explaining, as no original request or reminder to attend has been noted on your side.

Removing the emotion, you may start to sense that the pressure from the caller and requests for money are not what you would expect from someone working at the courthouse.

Responding in this new way, you can then take action from a place of seeking verification:

1.   Thank the caller, but explain you need to go and verify yourself before responding further
2.   Discontinue the call no matter how persistent the person on the phone is
3.   Double-check the story yourself with the court via a registered, official number

This is one example. For the other scams, you can consider how similarly diffusing the emotional reaction, the red flags start to appear.

For a different example, consider using elements of scams where you are offered something enticing (Mitten, 2017). Imagine you receive a call asking you to talk on stage at a conference along with a number of peers you admire. You accept the offer and add it to your calendar. A couple of weeks later you receive confirmation of the date and time you will be talking, in an email that also has an emotional plea as to whether you can cover some of the initial costs of hiring the venue – just until ticket sales are through. Removing the emotion (excitement at being asked to present at such an event), you may realise the payment request is abnormal, and that you should double-check and verify the event.

The examples in this chapter have been provided to start you thinking about how to unpack a story being told to you, so that if you are faced with any scam you might be able to identify it for what it is.

There is more information in the red flags checklist at the back of the book, including these high-level points to look out for:

•   **Abnormal behaviour**
•   **Pushy requests/time pressure** (but take note that fraudsters today are aware that this is a well-cited red flag, and some can be extremely patient!)
•   **Unusual payment methods suggested**
•   **Something simply does not make sense**
•   **Emotional conversation or content**

Action points

Each section in this chapter so far had its own advice. It was also constructed to build your overall ability to spot red flags and inconsistencies in general. The following are some overarching points to action before moving on to the summary of this chapter.

1. Add to your calendar to re-read this chapter in a year's time to refresh on how everyone is vulnerable to a well-packaged scam story
2. Make a commitment to be alert to any materials relevant professional bodies publish on any specific fraud attempts reported to them. For example, the BACP has produced a pamphlet "Scams: A Guide for Counsellors" (BACP, n.d.). The information in this guide would be currently applicable to other practitioners (coaches, therapists, psychologists)
3. Make a personal commitment to read alerts in the media or from authorities, going forward, and absorb what they are warning you about

Threat actors will change their modus as soon as they feel it has been exposed and can adapt their stories from one person to the next. This is why understanding the underpinnings of the fraud method and seeing the red flags will always be important.

In the event that you still become the victim of a scam of any kind, and find out after you have made a payment – use the "Action points if you become a victim of fraud" section in Chapter 7 to guide your first responses.

Summary

The human factor is a marked vulnerability in cybersecurity (Wiederhold, 2014). Much of the reason for this is arguably a lack of awareness and lack of ability to respond to either red flags or anything that might be suspicious. Each practitioner is a piece of their own cybersecurity puzzle.

The reflective exercises, alongside the concrete examples and the explanations, are there not only to build your knowledge, but also your ability to respond with awareness in the cyberspace.

Outcomes of this chapter include the following:

*   Awareness of scams that have been tailored to target your profession
*   Ability to unpack elements of a scam
*   Tips on how to avoid falling victim to scams
*   Information on how to spot and react to red flags

References

American Psychological Association Services, Inc. (2019, July 11). *More reports surface of telephone scammers targeting psychologists*. https://www.apaservices.org/practice /business/technology/telephone-scammers

Borders, J. (2019, November 22). *Active scam alert: Calls from people impersonating officers*. SacWellness. https://sacwellness.com/active-scam-alert/

Borders, J. (2021, August 21). *Currently active scams targeting therapists*. SacWellness. https://sacwellness.com/scams-targeting-therapists/

British Association for Counselling & Psychotherapy. (n.d.). *Scams: A guide for counsellors*. https://www.bacp.co.uk/about-us/contact-us/scams/

Button, M., Lewis, C., & Tapley, J. (2014). Not a victimless crime: The impact of fraud on individual victims and their families. *Security Journal*, *27*(1), 36–54. https://doi.org/10.1057/sj.2012.11

Caldwell, B. (2009, September 29). *Therapists targeted by spam, scams*. Ben Caldwell Labs. https://www.psychotherapynotes.com/?s=scam

Caldwell, B. (2019, December 4). Scams targeting health and wellness professionals (and how to avoid them). *SimplePractice*. https://www.simplepractice.com/blog/scam-alert/

Cavazos, J. (2018, November 20). *The jury duty scam you should know about*. ABC 10News. https://www.10news.com/news/national/the-jury-duty-scam-you-should-know-about

CPH & Associates. (n.d.). *Scam targeting therapists: What you need to know*. https://www.cphins.com/scam-targeting-therapist-what-you-need-to-know/

Furnell, S., & Shah, J. N. (2020). Home working and – an outbreak of unpreparedness? *Computer Fraud & Security*, *8*, 6–12. https://doi.org/10.1016/S1361-3723(20)30084-1

Gausden, G. (2020, April 18). Rise in fraudsters selling fake courses as more households take up online learning: We reveal five training scams and how to avoid them. This Is Money.co.uk. https://www.thisismoney.co.uk/money/beatthescammers/article-8213917/Rise-fraudsters-selling-fake-courses-reveal-five-online-training-scams.html

International Coaching Federation. (2020, October 20). *Reminder: Protecting your business from scams*. https://coachingfederation.org/blog/reminder-protecting-your-business-from-scams

Mitten, S. (2017, April 12). *Avoiding scams and shady deals targeting coaches*. International Coaching Federation. https://coachingfederation.org/blog/avoiding-scams-and-shady-deals-targeting-coaches

Pickup, O. (2020, September 7). Seven elearning scams to watch out for. *Raconteur*. https://www.raconteur.net/digital/online-learning-scams

United States Courts. (n.d.). Juror scams. https://www.uscourts.gov/services-forms/jury-service/juror-scams

Wade, C. (2018). *Teacher almost falls victim to potentially dangerous jury duty scam*. KTNV Las Vegas. https://www.ktnv.com/news/teacher-almost-falls-prey-to-jury-duty-scam

Warren-Hicks, C. (2020). Mental health counselor loses $6,000 to scam artists posing as Pensacola police. *Pensacola News Journal*. https://eu.pnj.com/story/news/crime/2020/08/10/scam-artists-posing-police-steal-6–000-pensacola-counselor/3319951001/

Wiederhold, B. K. (2014). The role of psychology in enhancing cybersecurity. *Cyberpsychology, Behavior, and Social Networking*, *17*(3), 131–132. https://doi.org/10.1089/cyber.2014.1502

Chapter 7

Payment fraud directed at your practice

Introduction

This chapter covers some of the payment fraud types and methods you are most likely to face in your practice that trick you into sending money to a fraudulent party. The previous chapter covered scams which can also lead to a payment being made, but the cases in this chapter have been separated for a reason. The scenarios in the next pages revolve around more direct routes to obtaining money from a victim, through fraudulent payment requests connected to something you might expect to pay (services/resources).

Loss of client data in these cases is usually rare; however, a reminder that fraud can lead to a complex aftermath. Experiencing fraud can mean an emotional time for victims, where they come to terms with what happened and why (Button et al., 2009). Financial losses can be accompanied by different feelings, reactions and emotions, from shame to disbelief. Clients may be affected by any business' downtime related to the fraud event; they may also become anxious as to whether the practice is secure enough and able to protect their identity. This is not to make you afraid but to make you aware why these are topics to take seriously. The threat of fraud is there, and it is not going away. It is lucrative business for cybercriminals.

The chapter does not cover all forms of payment fraud but filters to those the audience of this book may be most at risk of in their practices. By the end of this chapter, you will also have been introduced to how to reduce the risk of payment fraud occuring on your bank accounts and how to detect and act if payment fraud does occur.

The chapter will build the following:

Awareness

- of types of fraud that directly attempt to elicit a fictitious payment or re-route payment details of a genuine payment
- of how important it is to reconcile your bank accounts and check outgoing payments frequently

DOI: 10.4324/9781003184805-8

Understanding

of the need to double-check new payment details or unexpected invoices
of first steps – if you become a victim of fraud

Prevention tips and tricks

for preventing payment fraud occurring in your practice

*

Payment fraud directed at your practice

Payment fraud

Payment fraud is often described as unauthorised, false or illegal payments involving criminals. This is part of the view. More broadly explained, payment fraud can involve payments being made by a bank account holder, who has been deceived into making the payment, or by a third party via unauthorised access to an account. Examples of how payment fraud can be executed:

*   Via cards, browser based online banking payments, mobile app payments, other third-party payment services, cryptocurrency payments and any type of action involving payment of money to another
*   In person at a bank branch or over the phone with a bank
*   Person to person, for example, where a victim is tricked on the street into transferring money to another

We have already covered aspects of payment fraud a little in other chapters. Chapter 5 covered how criminals can obtain banking details and credentials through malware. In those cases, the criminals will typically execute the payments themselves, and the victim does not see this until later. Later in this chapter we will cover reconciling bank accounts, which can be a way account holders find irregular outgoing payments such as these. Chapter 6 illustrated scams targeted at practitioners that involve stories around their profession, where victims may subsequently execute payments to fraudsters. In this chapter, we turn, however, more specifically to payments targeted at your practices, involving, for example, fake business-as-usual payments, changes in banking details and unusual ad-hoc payments presented to a victim. We will unpack details of all of these in the next sections.

Business email compromise and email account compromise – including CEO fraud

As practitioners, you will be paying invoices for different services and tools you use in your business. Business email compromise (BEC), targeting business email accounts, and email account compromise (EAC), targeting individuals' emails accounts, involve victims responding to fraudulent/compromised emails and payment requests (FBI, n.d.).

This type of fraud relies heavily on the victim being tricked into believing a payment request or invoice is genuine or them not seeing red flags. Technology sets up the fraud attempt with any of: spoofing, use of a compromised email account, impersonation of company staff, deep fakes and falsified invoices, but completion is very much reliant on the human vulnerability factor. The victim makes the payment.

Key in BEC/EAC fraud is the following:

- Impersonation of a person or an entity you would expect to receive a payment request from – this could be someone from an authority (tax, government, other) or someone you work with
- Impersonation of a customer or a service provider, requesting return of money or payment for services rendered

The sub-types of this type of fraud that practitioners are most likely to face, with some contextual examples, are as follows:

Invoice fraud

- You receive an email from a supplier asking you to pay an invoice. You pay it and do not realise it was a fake invoice. Examples: fake invoices for services/resources – rent, marketing, other

Payment redirection fraud

- You receive a request to update payment details for a company/supplier you regularly pay invoices to. Later, the company calls you due to unpaid amounts; you discover that the payment details you were sent are fake and are redirecting payments you intended to your supplier to a fraudster. As you find this out quite late, your bank cannot retrieve any of the funds, and you still owe the actual company

CEO fraud

While this typically involves impersonation of the person at the top, practitioners have been targeted by variations of this involving spoofed members of professional bodies (APA, 2020). Here are examples of the elements of this type of fraud:

- The person who makes payments for your company receives a request from you or another person running your practice (a request you didn't write yourself) asking them to make a payment for a top-secret project you are working on or something specific the company "really needs". Remember social engineering – the packaging – typically the email will make the purchase sound like a really good win for the company, and the wording will thank the person making the payment in a way that makes them feel they are doing a great service to the company. The idea behind that is to elicit a positive emotional reaction in the person making the payment – that they feel they are part of achieving something great for the company and to encourage them to make the payment right away. It is only later that the person making the payment finds out that you didn't send the request – someone had hacked your email or spoofed it

- You go on a vacation, and when you return, one of the people working with you is happy to inform you that it's OK, they took care of the payment you forgot to make to a company you are working with on an important initiative. The problem is you hadn't forgotten anything, and there was no such initiative. Fraudsters knew you were out of town and got into action with a spoofed email
- A co-worker or a business partner asks you to make a payment towards something not totally unexpected, such as to return some money to another party, purchase something for the office or even purchase a number of gift cards (Royal Canadian Mounted Police [RCMP], n.d.). Again, social engineering often comes in here, with the co-worker having an emotive story such as they would do this themselves, but they aren't feeling too good, so it would be great if you can help out. You do so, not knowing your business partner's email was hacked (or spoofed), and they are not the one writing the email to you

Underlying methods fraudsters employ

Below are some examples. These fraud types are a very real threat, with evolving MOs (RCMP, n.d.; FBI, n.d.), so we will again in this chapter look at specific red flags that will help you spot other scenarios.

Invoice fraud and payment redirection fraud

1. The fraudster hacks into your company (or private) email account and finds invoices for services you typically pay for. A fake copy of an invoice is then created with the fraudster's own payment information on it. This is then sent to you from another email that may or may not be one spoofed to be similar to that of your supplier
2. The fraudster breaches a company that you receive regular invoices from (or have received an invoice from in the past). From there, they target customers of the company with fake invoices that they add their own payment information to
3. The fraudster engages in a mass phishing campaign. By targeting a large number of people, fraudsters inevitably will land with some who do use the product they are sending a fake invoice for
4. The fraudster targets you very specifically by researching upfront your practice, guessing or finding out which services you use and spoofing invoices for these

CEO fraud

1. The fraudster gains unauthorised access to your email account and from there issues a request (FBI, n.d.) to a colleague or an employee to make an important payment
2. Fraudsters spoof your email address to as close to the original as possible and then send emails to a colleague/employee asking them to make a payment (RCMP, n.d.). Your colleague doesn't pick up on the subtle differences of the spoofed email and makes the payment

The risk of BEC/EAC fraud

All sizes of companies are targeted. Medium to large-sized companies may pay more bills, giving the criminal more options to engineer payments out of unsuspecting staff (including for larger amounts) without much explanation.

Smaller businesses may make fewer payments but be equally susceptible through being unaware of this type of fraud (Jordan, 2019).

The APA (2020) and ICF (2019) have, for example, alerted that members have been targeted. All types of business can be. The elements pitched to match payments a business might expect to pay, to lure them in. The FBI produces a report annually on the basis of statistics from its Internet Crime Complaint Center. The 2020 report shows US$1.8 billion was lost in the United States to BEC and EAC. To further put the widespread threat of this fraud method into perspective: the total figure of losses reported to the FBI for internet and cybercrime complaints that same year was US$4.1 billion (Internet Crime Center, 2021). The FBI describes BEC and EAC fraud as financially one of the most damaging online crimes (FBI, n.d.).

BEC/EAC where your accounts have been compromised

If you fall victim to any of the scenarios depicted where someone has infiltrated your own systems, or due to malware, seek professional help and follow the steps in Chapter 5 in responding to a cyberattack.

How to mitigate it?

1. Know your suppliers! A key element of preventing this kind of fraud is knowing your suppliers (Met Police, 2014) and your expected outgoing payments

    *   If your supplier is located in Australia, and you receive new payment details for a bank in Poland, check it out

- If your supplier has always invoiced you on the last day of the month, but has this time sent one on the 14th, check it out
- For any request to pay ahead-of-time or earlier than an invoice date – ask questions, double check the payment you received and compare it to previous invoices
- If in any doubt at all – whether from seeing some red flags or just gut instinct – place a phone call to the company. Use the number you have always contacted them on. Do take time to corroborate requests you receive (Met Police, 2014)

2.   Match any suspicious invoices to previous invoices and correspondence you have had from the same place. In a spoofed invoice, some changes can be easy to spot if the fraudster is not very technical/experienced. Abnormalities to look for include accounting totals do not add up, margins have been altered, lines/boxes are formatted poorly and stamps/signatories are not quite in the same position. Numbers that need altering on an invoice – such as dates, invoice number, amount – are particularly fields a fraudster may have manipulated (Salmon, 2019). Check for irregular font size, style and spacing; also, sometimes, fraudsters forget to update one or the other of the fields. Most companies today use automated invoicing systems where all these small irregularities would not occur

3.   Take time to reflect on how these fraud types can affect your practice and what you can do about them. For example, if you have employees or co-workers who make payments for your practice, consider how you will train them on this information

4.   Remind your employees or anyone making payments for you that they can always check the authenticity of an invoice with you. Never show impatience or frustration with them when they do; instead, show gratitude that they are being vigilant. Keep a fully open door to anyone coming to you to do precisely that

5.   If fraudsters have gained access to a company's email account and have access to their billing system, formatting irregularities can be harder to spot. That is when it is important, on your side, to always check that the amount, services listed, invoice date, payment date are in line with expectations and to note, and investigate further, if there is any usual behaviour from that provider

New payee

- Whether you receive new bank account details before, or at the same time, as an invoice, check them thoroughly
- Check the bank account in an expected country – the first letters of an IBAN number, for example, indicate the country (IBAN, n.d.). This typically should match locations the company operates in; if not, ask questions

- When making a payment via your online banking system, do not ignore any alert that the payee name you have typed in does not match the name on the actual account. Ask questions, but always to the expected original supplier

New suppliers

Always also perform checks on any new company or supplier you work with or order from, particularly if you are responding to an advertisement or a flyer and the company is unknown to you. Things to check:

- Scrutinise the website, webshop content, formatting and style. Make sure you are not on a spoofed version of an original site. Spoofed sites may have a very subtle changes that you can pick up on
- Are their prices much lower than anywhere else, or does anything else sound too good to be true?
- Check for reviews of the company. If any red flags show, cross-check the company name by adding a term like "fraud" or "scam" to your search
- Images a company uses to sell its services/goods can be checked through a Google image search (https://images.google.com/) to see where else they show up. TinEye offers also a reverse image search (https://tineye.com/). These can help show if a company is using stock photos or whether the photos belong to a company they are spoofing

Identity theft

The notes on BEC/EAC fraud highlight areas where a practitioner's identity might be spoofed (CEO Fraud) or taken over. Prevention of any type of identity theft relies on the layers of security you have been encouraged already to implement. If you do want to find out more about identity theft, APA Services (2009) has produced a good guideline that covers what it is, how to mitigate it and what to do if it occurs. There are many other resources you can find online as well.

Key starter points to reduce the risk of your identity being stolen or someone impersonating you are as follows:

- Putting into place the defences you have already read about in the chapters up until now
- Spotting red flags and abnormal requests
- Not providing any sensitive personal information to another party
- Ensuring you are registered for any authority websites before someone else does it for you (Krebs, 2020)

- Taking care with the information about yourself or your company that you place online

Case study break – Delores

Now is a good time to take a break to read another full case study before reading on. Turn to the back of the book and look up "The Full Case of Delores" (p. 175). As with the other case studies, do take time to read it slowly and undertake the reflective elements to continue to build your skills and reactions.

Banking security basics

If you feel tempted to skim any of this section (or even others), don't forget that fraudsters are waiting for you. Remember, as noted in Chapter 1, they will target anyone, cybersecurity companies included (Mandia, 2020). The number of qualifications and competencies you have doesn't stop them. They see you as having data that can be sold, an income that can be exploited, and you likely have enough information online about yourself and your practice to get them started (Button et al., 2009).

If you are younger and have grown up with technology, don't assume that as giving you an edge either. Barclays conducted research that showed younger people with degrees appeared more susceptible to fraud, with one suggestion for this being their trust in technology (Boyce, 2017). Similarly, findings from Microsoft suggest that, when targeted with a tech support scam, both Gen Z and Millennials are more likely to continue to interact than other generations (Microsoft Stories Asia, 2021). As mentioned earlier, there is a story that can be told to any of you reading this book, that in the wrong time and place, you might fall for.

Do not give out credentials

When your bank, government or other sends messages reminding that they will never ask you for a pin or other code, this is actually true. Any company that runs anything you have access for does not need your credentials to look up your information. If you recall all the defence layers looked at in Chapter 2, on securing devices, those layers are yours alone. Any and all passwords, pins, MFA/2FA codes, memorable data – all the elements that are part of logging into something – are only needed by the person going in the front entrance or login screen of the product. That is, they are only needed by yourself. If you are thinking you have read this already in this book, the repetition is there because the public at large do not listen to this over and over again. Embed this into a core memory. Where you are ever asked for any of these credentials, your core memory, going forward, should issue a very large red flag in response.

Protecting bank accounts

The following information and actions are there to help protect your bank accounts. Much of this will also transfer to protecting your personal accounts as well as those you use for work. Remember to reframe the friction of any of the points and steps noted – they might prevent you from experiencing financial loss and the aftermath of being a fraud victim.

- Enable all banking security options available (MFA/2FA)
- Activate any account debit and balance alerts offered by your banking services. These are services where the bank sends an email or SMS when, for example, a payment over a set amount is made or an account balance goes under a set number
- Some banks also have a mobile banking app, where push messages pop up each time a payment is made. If they do, make full use of this feature
- Enable any maximum payment amount controls offered by your bank on accounts and cards. If anyone gains access to your accounts, they will then be limited as to what they can execute during a certain period of time. Giving you a possibility to potentially spot what is happening before they take all your money
- Check bank accounts regularly. It takes a couple of minutes to scan through your latest transactions. Never hesitate to check transactions with your bank that you cannot explain and do so as soon as possible
- If you are requiring a client to pay upfront, or have another reason to send banking information upfront to another party that you have not met or established a working relationship with, do your due diligence checks first, especially if it is a new client.
- Don't put banking information on your website
- While physical signatures add a nice visual touch to newsletters or other documents, evaluate whether what you are sending actually needs it. Consider creating a sign off using your practice name or your name in script but not a signature you have registered with banks or authorities
- Learn how your bank handles fraud disputes. Look up on their website or ask at your branch. Put any relevant phone numbers in your phone directory, but also keep them on paper, just in case a network or device becomes infected and unusable
- If you have a credit card (corporate/private) that you use infrequently, check if you have the ability to block it in your mobile banking when not in use. Some mobile banking apps allow you to block or freeze the card. Unfreezing/unblocking via the app is usually instantaneous and can be done just before you use it
- Don't be afraid to ask your bank how they are protecting your accounts. There is nothing wrong with ensuring that your bank has good track record with preventing fraud and doing a check if another bank has a better set-up

Liability

Some countries have legislation in place protecting the personal accounts of bank customers from fraud losses where the customer has not compromised their account credentials in any way. Check the specifics for your location, as this does change per country, with some having more liability with the bank (e.g. the United Kingdom) than others.

In the case of fraud loses on corporate accounts, typically, liability lies with the customer. Consider the following options if you have a corporate account:

- Review any corporate cyber liability insurance you have as to whether it extends to fraud losses
- Check if your bank offers banking insurance

Delegating banking to others

If you have someone help with your banking, do so via having a power of attorney or delegation agreement in place or set up a corporate account where you can give access to employees. This will ensure each person has their own login. Even if the person is a most-trusted close relative or a trusted employee, the following are some of the reasons to do this:

- If someone uses your credentials and fraud occurs, you may not be covered by the bank (where the account and case is one where the bank could be liable), as you have compromised your credentials to another party
- Banks often use security software that builds up a profile of the users logging-in, making it easier for them to detect abnormal login behaviour. So, having users log in using their own credentials may enable that the user builds a behavioural metric or analytic profile which the bank can use towards keeping your account safe
- People are likely to be more responsible for their own login credentials, as their actions can be traced back to them

---

Incoming payments and client names

Note that someone you delegate bank account access to will see the names of clients you have on the incoming amounts. Have you aligned this to how you operate your practice and how your clients are informed on who has knowledge of their identity?

Action points if you become a victim of fraud

The following is a list of suggested initial steps if you believe you have become the victim of payment fraud. Please note that where you have become a victim due to malware or any form of infiltration of your systems, follow the action steps in Chapter 5 primarily, with these as supplementary. Do follow advice from your bank and authorities as well as this list, as it is not exclusive. Depending on your location and the fraud that has been committed, you may be required to follow more steps.

- **Call** your bank. Many have a 24-hour helpline for fraud reporting. They can help with blocking cards, accounts and other. If a payment has only recently left your account, the sooner you call the bank, the more chance there is they can recover it
- If your bank does not have a 24-hour helpline, and it is out of hours, check what is on their website. Change your passwords and block any cards that you can freeze yourself. If you have become a victim due to malware, remember not to do this from an infected device or network!
- Some banks will offer that you can make a dispute online. Do this if the phone lines are out of hours. The best thing to do is phone in still once the bank is open. Having a conversation with someone there, you will understand better what can be done to protect your accounts as well as attempt to recall payments. The longer you take to report a payment as fraud, the lesser the chance that the money will be recovered
- Make a police report. Your bank will also guide you to do this if they need this for the case you open with them

Practitioner versus cybersecurity expert

In this section let's briefly cover how the skills that you have when operating as a coach, therapist, counsellor or other practitioner can potentially make you extra vulnerable to the scenarios presented in Chapters 6 and 7.

The audience reading this book are in professions where they often support the people they work with from a place of unconditional positive regard (Standal, 1954). This human factor that supports your profession can be a problem when it comes to cybersecurity. As well as being the supportive professional your clients are looking for, in order to protect those clients and your practice from cyber-criminals, you need to also have a side that can be sceptical. For example, when not in session with a client and being told a story by someone you do not know, claiming to be x informing you about y, you need to put way the unconditional positive regard. As practitioners, you can however re-utilise your competencies in listening, querying and being curious. These may prove optimal qualities in your role of creating a solid defence line as the "human firewall" (Osterman Research, 2018, p. 16) of your security set-up against cybercrime and fraud.

You are trained in being able to help your clients unpack many topics, and show understanding and empathy in addition to being good listeners. Fraudsters are after inducing emotional responses in their victims. Some of their scams will appeal to your nature to help others. Others may arouse fear through pressure or a threat against your practice. Reflect on strategies you believe would keep you level-headed in such a situation – what would work for you to remember you are not talking to a client? How can you ensure always to dig into the elements of a story being unfolded – with the scepticism noted earlier until proven otherwise?

Cartoonist John Klossner (2006) depicts the challenge in a cartoon posted on his website. It shows a boxing ring. The ringmaster announces that, in one corner, there are a number of cyber defences, and in the other corner, there is Dave. The idea being that no matter how many prevention tools a person has, it just takes one human to open the door. As illustrated in this chapter, some types of fraud need you as the human factor for them to be executed. Thus, in your cybersecurity set-up, your role is as important as the technological defences you put in place.

Consider building a contingency plan for what you would do if you did experience a cyber event or fraud incident of any kind (Met Police, 2014). Remember to keep a copy of the plan printed offline. This can apply whether you are a sole entrepreneur or whether you employ staff.

Summary

This was the last of three chapters looking at particular threats practitioners face. The chapters have aimed to provide information in a way that the elements of the threats are clear, so that however they are packaged, a practitioner may pick up on them.

In this chapter, methods of manipulating another into making a payment were discussed. Outcomes have included the following:

• Understanding the benefit of thoroughly reviewing invoices before going ahead and paying them
• Looking for red flags in unusual payment requests
• Tips on how to carefully review changes to beneficiaries' banking information
• First steps in response if fraud occurs
• Importance of checking bank accounts and card transactions on a regular basis

You are now better armed to spot red flags and anomalies, and mitigate the risk of cybercrime. Where something still occurs, you are now also more ready to react and know some of the first steps to take. Chapter 8 will tie up elements of data, ethics and cybersecurity from a more practical, client-facing view before the book then rounds up with some extra checklists and final thoughts.

References

American Psychological Association. (2020, March 11). *How to avoid email scams*. https://www.apa.org/about/division/digest/share-members/avoid-email-scams

American Psychological Association Services Inc. (2009, April 30). *Identity theft: Take steps to minimize your risk.* https://www.apaservices.org/practice/update/2009/04-30/identity-theft

Boyce, L. (2017, May 8). *Young people with degrees are the banking customers most likely to be duped by online fraudsters, shock new research.* This Is Money.co.uk. https://www.thisismoney.co.uk/money/beatthescammers/article-4484396/Those-degree-education-likely-fall-scams.html

Button, M., Lewis, C., & Tapley, J. (2009). *Fraud typologies and the victims of fraud: Literature review.* National Fraud Authority. https://assets.publishing.service.gov.uk/government/uploads/system/uploads/attachment_data/file/118469/fraud-typologies.pdf

FBI. (n.d.). *Business email compromise.* https://www.fbi.gov/scams-and-safety/common-scams-and-crimes/business-email-compromise

Google. (n.d.). *Google images.* https://images.google.com/

IBAN. (n.d.). *IBAN validation and calculation.* https://iban.com

International Coaching Federation. (2019, October 31). *Email fraud alert.* https://coachingfederation.org/blog/email-fraud-alert

Internet Crime Center. (2021). *Internet crime report 2020.* FBI. https://www.ic3.gov/Media/PDF/AnnualReport/2020_IC3Report.pdf

Jordan, A. (2019, March 26). *Invoice fraud: Many small businesses aren't aware of the risks.* SmallBusiness.co.uk. https://smallbusiness.co.uk/supplier-fraud-real-risk-protect-business-2543085/

Klossner, J. (2006). Human security. *J. Klossner Cartoons.* https://www.jklossner.com/

Krebs, B. (2020, August 12). *Why and where you should plant your flag.* Krebs on Security. https://krebsonsecurity.com/2020/08/why-where-you-should-you-plant-your-flag/

Mandia, K. (2020, December 8). FireEye shares details of recent cyber attack, actions to protect community. *Fire Eye.* https://www.fireeye.com/blog/products-and-services/2020/12/fireeye-shares-details-of-recent-cyber-attack-actions-to-protect-community.html

Met Police. (2014). *The little book of big scams.* https://www.met.police.uk/SysSiteAssets/media/downloads/central/advice/fraud/met/little-book-of-big-scams-business-edition.pdf

Microsoft Stories Asia. (2021, July 22). *Tech support scams remain a threat globally and in Asia Pacific despite drop in encounters: Microsoft survey.* Microsoft. https://news.microsoft.com/apac/2021/07/22/tech-support-scams-remain-a-threat-globally-and-in-asia-pacific-despite-drop-in-encounters-microsoft-survey/

Osterman Research. (2018). *Best practices for protecting against phishing, ransomware and email fraud – an Osterman research white paper.* https://www.agari.com/advanced-threat-protection/analyst-research/osterman-best-practices-protecting-email-attacks.pdf

Royal Canadian Mounted Police. (n.d.). *Business email compromise (BEC).* https://www.rcmp-grc.gc.ca/en/business-email-compromise-bec

Salmon, J. (2019, April 8). 15 steps to avoid invoice fraud. *The Credit Protection Association.* https://www.cpa.co.uk/15-steps-to-avoid-invoice-fraud/

Standal, S. (1954). *The need for positive regard: A contribution to client-centered theory* (Unpublished doctoral dissertation). University of Chicago, Department of Psychology.

TinEye. (n.d.). *Reverse image search.* https://tineye.com/

Chapter 8

Ethics and data

Introduction

The professions this book is aimed at typically have confidentiality at the heart of any client relationship and a desire to provide services that can change the lives of those they work with. As shown previously, that is challenging when working in a world with an ever-growing cyber footprint, where criminals are waiting in line to exploit weaknesses.

This chapter ties together elements from the rest of the book identifying some of a practitioner's day-to-day actions required to keep data secure and aligning these actions with ethical codes of conduct. Topics covered include how to actually secure data (including storage and backups), anonymising/deidentifying data, informing clients about cyber risks and setting boundaries on transmission over networks.

The following pages will show the deeper connection of cybersecurity to ethics and data and provide practical advice and guidance that cannot be readily accessed elsewhere. The message for the reader throughout this chapter is that data security, cybersecurity and ethics are inextricably linked. Cybersecurity enables data security, which underlies the ethics and confidentiality expectations from clients when they seek services/help from your professions.

Outcomes at the end of the chapter:

Enhanced knowledge

New appreciation and understanding of why data protection/privacy laws exist
Deeper understanding of the connection between cybersecurity, ethics and
   protecting data

Practical applications

Tips on securing client records
Information on data storage options

DOI: 10.4324/9781003184805-9

New competences and behaviours

Confidence to be open and transparent with clients about cyber risks

Ability to confidently contract/inform clients regarding your data security protocols

Confidence to explain the cybersecure space you have created

Ability to inform clients on their role in keeping your shared interactions safe

*

Ethical guidelines

Professional bodies and personal responsibility

The term "professional bodies" will be used for ease of reference to cover the variety of professional membership bodies, licencing boards and associations that many practitioners take steps to be accredited, licenced or associated with. Professional bodies have frameworks that often include competency requirements and ethical codes that their members are expected to adhere to. Professional bodies have not been without critique. Not all countries have introduced statutory requirements for professionals – in the United Kingdom, for example, there is a lack of regulation of counsellors and psychotherapists (BACP, 2020). Similarly, accreditation frameworks for coaching have come under criticism for being neither evidence based nor validated extensively (Griffiths & Campbell, 2008) and lacking regulation. This fact appears to be inspiring newer initiatives such as the British Psychological Society creating a coaching psychology chartership pathway (Stopforth, 2019). Overall, depending on their location, profession and level of training, a practitioner may or may not be subject to any statutory national regulatory requirements.

Even in the most basic of trainings, safeguarding clients and confidentiality are topics that consistently come up. However, due to the fact that professional bodies are often not regulated, nor have overarching expectations put upon them from governmental bodies, elements of their competency frameworks and their ethics codes tend to be carefully worded when it comes to what is expected and what is actually *enforceable* on a member. Members are though, expected to see them as binding and abide by them; they are informed of the consequences if they are found to not do so.

Many working as coaches, therapists, psychologists or counsellors are then individually responsible for ensuring due ethical care in respect of their clients. This is where national-level data protection and privacy legislation can be seen as having very positive effects. Across all professions and levels of training, practitioners are obliged to adhere to government-level laws and regulation.

This book similarly cannot enforce cybersecurity on you as the reader, but it has tackled the gap of some of the practical steps which can be applied to help secure the cyberspace used by you and your clients, which is currently missing in other guidelines. It has also reinforced throughout how cybersecurity is essential when it comes to ensuring client confidentiality, data security and protecting your practice from cybercrime. Although separate concepts, cybersecurity and data protection are inextricably linked and apply equally to very complex systems as they do to the humble email, zoom call, spreadsheet and word document.

Grouping where standards come from

Four groups sum up many of the areas that practitioners turn to when it comes to standards expected from them:

1. National law, and also local law in larger countries with local area governance
2. Guidelines, codes, standards and competency frameworks created by professional bodies (accreditation bodies, associations, licencing boards, professional membership organisations)
3. Guidelines, policies, requirements created by the companies, school systems or other industry bodies that a practitioner may come in contact with – or form a working relationship with
4. Personal standards and values, perhaps informing our decision-making and behaviours around ensuring laws or other professional standards are acted upon and upheld

Group 1: national/local law is the group that is most enforceable through fines and penalties, where lack of application of the legislation can be proved. Group 3: guidelines from parties you work with can be very specific, and each practitioner will need to scrutinise these as applicable to them.

Returning to Group 2: while many professional bodies may lack an enforcement role, there are many still positives to mention. They have enabled the professions to become more consistent. When applying and renewing membership of a body, it would be difficult for a member to hide if they do not have the necessary competencies or do not apply ethics as stated (a disclaimer that there have been cases of scam practitioners, perhaps stories for another edition). Many professional bodies also state clearly that a breach of ethics can be used towards evaluating complaints made against a member.

Some non-accredited practitioners and practitioners-in-training still opt to adhere to the ethical practices of one of these bodies even if they do not apply for accreditation, as they provide a solid ethical framework that they can abide by and inform their clients they follow.

Many professional body competency frameworks or ethics codes, at the time of writing, do mention data security. They just do not, yet, bring up practical competences around securing data or any expectations around cybersecurity. For example, the ICF (2019) reverts members to relevant laws when it comes to securing data and states as a competency: "maintains confidentiality with client information per stakeholder agreements and pertinent laws" (Competency A.1.5., p. 1).

Practitioners, then, are often clear from legislation that they need to be aware of topics such as data security, data processing, data storage, data deletion and data breaches. They are often also referred to the same data legislation or provided re-writes of it in more digestible forms by professional bodies. They are not, however, provided with clear information on the practical side of achieving this. So far this book has covered much around the practical side to securing data, and the next pages take on data storage, deletion and anonymisation to close out some remaining topics brought up in legislation and ethics frameworks.

This "practical" side is important, as without cybersecure practices and behaviours, a practitioner cannot fulfil the points in ethical guidelines where they are called to "respect the dignity and worth of the individual" (European Association of Psychotherapy [EAP], Statement of Ethical Principles, 2018, p. 1). To achieve this, you need to handle clients' data through protecting it carefully. As you have seen through the previous chapters, cybercriminals don't operate using the same guidelines; they are not concerned about what will happen to your clients' dignity and worth if they sell their data on the darknet.

As written by the American Counselling Association (ACA) (2014):

> Trust is the cornerstone of the counseling relationship, and counsellors have the responsibility to respect and safeguard the client's right to privacy and confidentiality.

To really take ethical responsibility to protect a client's privacy and confidentiality in today's technological world, where cybercriminals will exploit any weakness they can find, Group 4 – of personal standards – is key.

In order to mitigate the harm, distress or other negative outcome from a data breach or cyber incident, it is the responsibility of each practitioner to ensure that their practice is as cybersecure as possible through the following:

- Confidential processing, storage and deletion of client records/traces – towards a reduction in harm and impact on clients, from any exfiltration, deletion or alteration of records during a cyber incident
- Ensuring secure storage of records for the required period of time expected of a practitioner for good record-keeping and to enable correct and suitable treatment/services for of a client
- Ensuring secure exchange of information, data and safe communications
- Protecting the practice itself from the harm of a cyber event, scam or fraud, which can have a follow-on effect of hindering future interactions with clients and reputational damage

These points are necessary to mitigate harm to the client from the impact of their innermost world being exposed. Also more simply you have explicitly offered confidentiality as part of your service; so now it's time to ensure it.

By now, you are more prepared than you probably realise. Many of the activities in the book, now put into action, have helped you ensure you are on the way to achieving the aforementioned. Cybercriminals wait for open doors and take opportunities without question, so keeping the doors that are in your control closed is proactive, preventative and essential. It is a little similar to considering ethical dilemmas when working with clients. We can look back at them retroactively, or choose to look at them proactively (Hirani, 2017). That a cyberattack can result in loss of data, loss of reputation, business downtime and a financial hit should mean everyone is proactive in protecting and securing their systems and the client data they contain.

Before returning to topics around data later in this chapter, we will take a time-out and thereafter look at how you can talk to clients about how you secure your practice. An explanation of your cybersecurity practices will help you stand out as a practitioner who takes care and pride in considering client confidentiality (ideas on how to do this are provided). It demonstrates you have evaluated broader aspects of safety when it comes to the client. In a world where data privacy, data breaches and GDPR are not new topics for anyone, this will be noticed.

*

A mindfulness time-out

There will be moments when legislation, laws, privacy/data protection and ethics feel like overwhelming topics: either you feel under pressure to "get it right" or it feels overwhelming when you simply just want to run a business to help people. The below exercise combines elements of mindfulness and self-compassion – both of which have been shown to have positive benefits to psychological health (Ivtzan & Lomas, 2016).

Acceptance

Become present with any frustration and spend a minute to have some self-compassion for having to navigate a complex world that you probably have not received any or a lot of training for. The law, regulation and consequences are very rarely part of any training courses a practitioner has undertaken. Accept and forgive yourself for how you are feeling. Recognise you are not alone and take a moment to absorb that others in your profession will be feeling the same way.

Reset

While frustrating, legislation is extremely important. Some argue that just as access to the internet may become a human right, so to could cybersecurity (Shackelford, 2019). As practitioners (or any service provider), you do need to hold client data to be able to provide services; the balance is in learning to be cybersecure and protect a person's privacy.

Start again: consider if you were your client. Reframe also how much your clients might appreciate your efforts to keep their data secure. With anything you have not yet done or researched, make a short plan of small, realistic steps. Put them on your calendar.

Visualisation exercise

Picture your dream castle. Imagine your dream castle is in an area where it can come under attack. Now consider the castle as your business. Walking around the grounds are people. They are your clients.

Ensure your castle has a solid drawbridge and guards. Add windows high up the walls, with sentries looking out. Consider how else you want to defend it? A second wall around the grounds? A moat?

Deep inside the castle, visualise the library. The library is where you store all your data. How secure is the library door? How many locks are on it? Are there other ways in?

*

Cybersecurity contracting with clients

Most professional bodies encourage the practitioner/member to contract with clients on all aspects of how they will work together. The Global Code of Ethics (2021) adopted by the Association of Coaching (AC) and the European Mentoring & Coaching Council (EMCC), among other professional bodies, notes that in contracting, clarity is made of all aspects of how the coach and client will work together, including "logistics". The BACP (2018) has similar guidance in their Ethical Framework for the Counselling Professions and makes it clear that, in contracting, clarity can be provided to the client on how their confidentiality and privacy will be upheld.

Contracting often includes giving clients information on which code of conduct/ethics the practitioner adheres to and the professional bodies they belong to, perhaps with a short explanation of how this ensures they have met certain competencies. While not practical to go through every item of the competencies/ ethics codes with clients, confidentiality is typically one of the topics always brought up. This makes contracting the ideal place to strengthen the trust you establish with a client, through briefly explaining some fundamental security essentials you have in place to safeguard your clients and their data. Making your security transparent demonstrates the time and effort you put into this to your client; it can also help keep you accountable to it.

Activity

Open your reflective notes.
The following exercise is to generate thinking around your own practice; there are no right or wrong answers.

Consider some of the case studies you have read plus the chapters on video conferencing and cyberthreats. Now that you have this knowledge, reflect and document your thoughts on the following:

Where do you want to place your boundaries on requests from clients on how to connect together and operate?

As you reflect, bring to mind all of the four groups mentioned in the previous section and how these may impact on your answer. In other words, the influence of legislation requirements, professional body expectations, the policies (or other) of any third party you work with, and finally how you yourself want to operate ethically.

Some prompts (should you need them):

- Reverting to your new knowledge from Chapter 4 on online communication and the case story with Delores, does this influence how you want to contract, going forward, in relation to communications tools and data shared via such tools?
- How do you personally want to make visible the steps you take to keep your practice as cybersecure as possible?
- If you were your client, what do you think you would like to hear?

Complete your reflections before reading further.

Importance of this exercise

Alongside setting steps to enable a more cybersecure practice, it can also be useful and important to reflect on where the lines are for a practitioner. If a client pushes to interact, for example, over an insecure media, how will you respond? Are you ready to provide a clear, professional response related to data security and risks in the cyberspace? Being able to reflect and bring into consideration a wider view, including different perspectives and positions, may mean a practitioner takes a proactive decision, ensuring taking a "mature attitude" to ethical dilemmas (Hirani, 2017, p. 12). This might also be important around data, where practitioners do not want to lose clients but may need to set boundaries where they have a client wanting to communicate or share information as follows:

- In a way the practitioner is not comfortable with
- Over an insecure service
- Not within the boundaries of law/legislation

- In a way that puts the practitioner, client or others at risk
- Other factor(s)

Finally, if you are also a client of a coach or therapist yourself, as well as a practitioner, consider turning the tables and consider how the information in this book may have made you also think differently about how your own data is stored by others. Does that make you more aware to ask questions when you are a client? Reflecting from this view, does this bring up any considerations towards how you want your own clients to feel or what you want them to know?

Ethics codes and data privacy laws are there to enable people to ask questions about what happens to their data, gain answers and feel they have more awareness and control over who has access to their data and how it is processed, protected and eventually deleted. Often this part is forgotten, as the focus tends to switch to implementation and avoiding penalties and issues, rather than the original purpose behind legislation.

Informing clients

Having a long conversation about cyber risks and mitigation at the contracting stage is, however, neither practical nor what is being recommended here. Some of you reading this will already have information for clients on your implementation of data privacy legislation, and this may be somewhere you can add some of the finer points or details. Consider also including details on your practices to secure client data and your boundaries on data sharing into contracts or terms of service. Ensure still to refresh on the main points you choose to make in verbal contracting and at any other relevant point in your relationship with the client.

Note your clients don't need to know precisely all the (procedural) detail of how you store and protect their data. It would be ill-advised to put precise details in writing that if in the hands of a criminal could enable them to find your client data or records or breach your security protections. Consider the following example: regarding secure storage of data, your clients just need to know that you have put in solid cybersecurity around your practice to protect data, that you only use tools you have researched as trusted, and that you keep yourself informed and updated on new cyber risks. They don't need to know how you save documents, name them, or add passwords to them.

Explaining elements of what you do is positive and a selling point for your practice.

Here is an example:

> *This practice uses tool ABC for any and all online calls/interactions. This software has been selected as it is currently one of the most secure conferencing tools. It should be noted that, with any internet-based tool and also any storage of data (e.g. notes from our sessions), there is always a small risk of a data breach. However, this practice has implemented a number of*

cybersecurity best practices and regularly re-reviews its cybersecurity and the tools used to ensure as trusted an environment as possible.

A final tip: know your client. A practitioner is only able to control how they handle data on their side. There is also a copy on the side of the sender of what they have sent and received. So, always consider whether you know your client well enough to know if they are likely to make a good decision regarding the transmission, storage and eventual deletion of information, chats, emails. If they will not, take this into consideration.

*

Data

So far, we have looked through the chapters on different aspects of data handling, such as transmission, and technical security around its storage. This section will round out some points on data storage from a more administrative viewpoint and the important connection to cybersecurity and legislation.

Legislation

Law and regulation around privacy and data (such as GDPR, other country regulations) are covered in countless books, trainings and materials. It is important that readers refer to the applicable resources on any such legislation, adhere to them and take legal advice as needed. What will be added here is practical information on topics that come up. Information and practical ideas and tips on how to actually keep data safely stored, retained and why deletion is necessary will be provided. This not only is pertinent to achieving what is required by legislation but continues the theme of cybersecurity around the data you process and store. This adds a final data-care layer on top of all the defence layers actioned through the chapters, aiding towards that the data contained behind those defences is as protected as possible.

Handling client data

At this stage, you may have started to form questions such as how to store the actual data files concerning clients in your practice? From the legislative/regulatory/practitioner perspective, it is important you turn to several different resources to answer this, which may include the following:

- The ethics guidelines of any accreditation bodies, supervision authorities or professional bodies and societies you belong to and follow
- If you reside in the EU, the applied GDPR regulation in the country (or countries) in which you operate and within which you store client data
- Any data privacy/protection or other applicable laws of the country (or countries) in which you operate, including all countries you store client data in

- Any other authority or body you are accountable to, for your practice and line of work
- For researchers, the guidelines laid down by the researching ethics boards you submit your research proposals to

If you reside or operate in multiple countries, you may need to take legal advice regarding this as professional bodies are not always clear in what this will mean. For example, from the coaching Global Code of Ethics (2021) the practitioner's responsibilities include the following:

> *Safe and secure maintenance of all related records and data that complies with all relevant laws and agreements that exist in their country regarding data protection and privacy.*
>
> (p. 7)

The term "their country" is a little undefined (as to if this is work, residential or both). Check the ethics codes you follow for equivalent constructions, and what they will mean for your situation and practice. As needed, ask your professional body for more clarity.

If you are in the EU, GDPR is a primary regulation. The guidance of the local data protection commissioner on certain points is also key. It is also important to refer to all relevant legislation for your country/countries. If you are not in the EU, you still need, as a practitioner who holds confidential client data, to be aware of any equivalent data protection laws and privacy laws in your country/countries. As a starting point, reach out to any associations and bodies you belong to, as they may have a full list of what applies to your particular profession in your location. Example internet searches you can do if you want to double-check yourself:

Data protection legislation in XYZ (add your country)
Privacy laws for customer/client data in XYZ (add your country)

Bear in mind that if you have clients from various countries, they may themselves have expectations around data security based on requirements in their own countries. Therefore, when you discuss data security during the contracting process, you can always confirm with them their understanding of this and whether they have any concerns.

While professional bodies tend to repeat the contents of laws or regulations to avoid any mis-advice to professionals, it is still worth looking up what they have written. Many of you will have done this. For those who haven't, here are some examples that may provide an idea of what to look for in terms of your profession, location and relevant associations/professional bodies.

The British Psychological Society (2018) has a compact version of GDPR, for example, and further refers readers to the Information Commissioner's Office (ICO) for more support. The ICO has a full suite of further explanations on data protection, including a guide to GDPR (ICO, n.d.). BACP (n.d.), provides some advice on applying GDPR to its members. Again, the wording highlights that practitioners need to consider all aspects of law and situations applicable to themselves, but the explanations may be useful. The ICO Guidance also provides useful information on pseudonymisation and anonymisation and the minimum period for retaining documents pertaining to a client.

Remember that legislation on securing data protects you as well as your clients; a data breach may damage your reputation and could result in financial penalties and costs.

Training providers

A side note for practitioners providing training or courses: remember to check any legislation on the length of time you can store data on participants and whether you need to disclose this to participants as part of the course information. When creating your course, consider what measures you can implement to avoid fake practitioners taking your courses or someone paying another person to take a course in their place (especially where you have no video contact or 1:1 time to prove otherwise). Also be alert to anyone changing their name once a training certificate is ready for them (training platforms do not always have controls to prevent it). If you run courses with hundreds/thousands of participants, there will be other challenges to consider. Where you have a high number of participants, it is well worth seeking an appropriately qualified consultant to assist with course protections and secure maintenance of participant data, including payment information.

Secure data retention

A data breach can occur from a cyberattack, as outlined in earlier chapters, and also from careless or inadequate handling of data, where data is exposed to someone who is not permitted to have access to it.

As noted earlier in this chapter, most ethics guidelines, codes of practice, advice from professional bodies have default statements reverting the practitioner to respect data storage and handling in line with legislation and regulation in the relevant country. They don't, however, cover what constitutes applicable data and how to actually secure it. This section will look at some of the types of data you may hold in your practice and offer tips on how to securely store it.

Data sets

Client static data

This is data about your client that includes their name and contact information. Depending on how you keep records, it may include other demographics.

Client background data

This is information about a client's background that you may document when first engaging with them This may include information from anyone referring the client or information sent by the client themselves.

Client session data

This involves the notes and information taken within an individual session.

Calendar records

These include appointments recorded in calendars and invitation details sent by a calendar app, booking tool, email or video conferencing tool.

Logs

Overarching logs of all coaching hours, kept for fulfilling record-keeping requirements or for accreditation purposes.

Conversations

These are emails, chats and other written correspondence. Verbal conversations are normally live/real time and not typically "data" unless intercepted by a threat actor recording passively or where some practitioners take a recording for specific purposes (either for training purposes or providing to the client) or where the practitioner writes up and sends notes afterwards.

Client invoices and payment records

These include payment records on your bank account/payment receipts held for accounting purposes showing the name of the client; also, invoices created and sent to clients stored for accounting purposes.

To start unfolding a very important point: while criminals can potentially cause the most harm through obtaining and exposing session records, your peripheral data records (such as calendar entries, invoices, receipts) are those that can be used to reidentify and expose client names where the names on session records have been anonymised. Peripheral records can alone expose a practitioner's client list. For some clients, just having their name exposed might be enough to cause harm, where they want to/have reasons to keep their participation in therapy/counselling/coaching/other entirely private.

Activity

Open your reflective notes and take an honesty check:

- Evaluate how you retain data in each of the aforementioned data sets
- How secure is your handling of the data in these data sets?
- When and how are you deleting the data in these data sets?
- Are there any data sets you cannot delete?

Data deletion

Each reader will have answered these reflections differently. Each data set can offer an exposure point if the data is not handled adequately or securely. For the last activity point, you will have noted that there are some records a practitioner does not have control over to delete, such as bank records. However, many banks will, after some years, archive records and they are themselves subject to data legislation. What you can control at all times is who has access to all data sets and when those in your control are deleted, after record-keeping requirements are fulfilled. For example, if someone has access to your bank accounts or booking calendar, is this known by your clients? Are those with access aware of confidentiality around your client base?

Practitioners using systems/software to hold data

If you use particular systems or software in your practice for bookings, storing client data and session notes, invoicing and accounts, CRMs/marketing, then you need to, per advice earlier in the book, always use best-in-class products that have security as a core part of their set-up.

Third-party tools can be breached at any time. To give an example, in December 2021, a ransomware attack hit a company that supplies systems supporting (among others) private practitioners, including psychologists (Lorenzen, 2022).

Your clients are only as protected as both the quality and security of the product you use and your cybersecurity set-up around it. How many clients' names and matching contact details would someone find in your accounting system, for example? The advice coming next applies largely to manually held data, but you can consider how to adapt it to your use of systems.

Keeping data safer

Author's view

Client data is essential, but it also reveals who you are working with. The traditional advice to anonymise files goes a short distance in a world where cybercriminals can gain full access to your computer.

With full access to your computer and programmes, I could demonstrate fairly quickly how easy it is to identify your clients (or reidentify them if they are anonymised). Here are some examples: I would search files with key terms such as: client, log, records, reflection, invoices, receipts, banking, accounting, see what I find and go deeper from there. A practitioner's calendar also reveals much: names, email addresses and perhaps notes. Names and email addresses can be used in searches through email accounts and other files.

The time and date of a calendar event or meeting might be something I can correlate to the last saved/modified date of client records or logs to discover which records correlate to which client – discovering the alias that has been used for a client. Alternatively, with access to accounting records, I can see the dates invoices are issued for or the receipts sent. Each of these records revealing names of clients which again might be correlated back to logs created or saved on similar dates.

Disconnecting data sets

It may be clearer now why protecting our cyber space requires a layered approach to security, including the actions and suggestions throughout this book. Each layer makes it harder for someone to gain unauthorised access into our devices, accounts and data. Whilst difficult as noted in the previous section to prevent someone piecing together who your clients are, from the data they find, there are ways you can make it much more complex to do so. Here are some starter suggestions, as you read, consider other ideas of your own:

1. Continue, as you likely do now, to write up background information and session logs pertaining to clients with an alias name. Remember to never store any client static data (name, address) in these files. Do not use an alias that includes their initials or other identifying data. You are strongly recommended to password protect these core documents and store them separately from any other records pertaining to your practice
2. Avoid, if possible, to put the date and session time in the session logs noted in point 1. This is because it will matter very little that you gave your clients an alias if a hacker can correlate the date and time on your session logs to your calendar invitations, (where you likely have your client's email address and therefore information that can identify them)
3. Some professional bodies require you keep records with the date and time of your sessions. Consider how you can keep this separately in an overarching log of your hours, which you store in a very different place to your client background information and session logs. You are strongly recommended to password protect this core document
4. Get creative on how you will remember which client you gave which alias name to
5. Consider how you can save all your client files in a way that doesn't draw attention to them. Is there a naming system that will draw less attention to them than: "Client List 2022" under "Business"? The more professional criminal can and will do more advanced searches into your individual documents, but a less experienced and equipped criminal may find it hard to find anything useful through the maze of documents you have gathered over time on your device
6. Do not share a device with client-related information with anyone, including your own family and colleagues. No matter how much you trust someone, they should not be anywhere near your client data! If you are in a situation

where you need, for any reason, to share with others a computer with client data on it (not recommended), some operating systems will enable you to have more than one login account. Set this up for anyone else who needs to use the same device as a very minimum and set boundaries on what they can add to your computer. Remove the added account as soon as its purpose has passed and see this as a solution for emergencies only. Additionally, do not let another person take that device with them to a location you are not aware of

Depending on the sophistication of a criminal who has taken your data, they may still connect the dots whatever you do, but you can make it harder for them to do so in case your data is compromised.

Practitioners working for other companies

Ensure you implement and comply with the company's cybersecurity policy. If they do not have one, you can use this guidance to discuss with them how you would like to operate securely.

Data deletion

Many practitioners, proud of their track record of working a number of hours with clients, might be tempted to keep records longer than required to by professional bodies/licensing boards or longer than permitted by data legislation. Whilst tempting to assume you keep data longer by removing names, please take great care with this. It is not always easy to fully remove any and all possible ways to trace data back to a person. If you are required to delete after a set number of years, the advice here is: just do it. Remember also to delete across each of the aforementioned data sets and any others you have.

Don't be afraid to have data!

Cyberattacks and data laws can potentially make practitioners nervous and concerned about having data. It is a natural reaction to feel concerned about holding data for a number of years knowing the threats that are out there. The reason you have read this book and implemented the layers of defence brought up so far is precisely to keep your data as secure as possible. Handling and storing data is an extremely necessary part of a practitioner's day-to-day operations. Importantly, as well as there being legislation around data protection, there is also legislation expecting many of the professionals reading this book to retain data for a minimum period of time.

Enabling you to keep data secure is at the heart of this book, as is enabling you to do this on an ongoing basis and being able to show that you have diligently done everything you can to protect your clients. Nothing in this book is here to suggest that you should not record client data or minimise what you record or hold.

To create value for your clients, data is necessary!

Most practitioners will be required to keep accurate, sufficient client records for some of the following reasons. Depending on your exact profession, there may be others you can add.

- Requirements at legislative level (national/local law and regulations)
- Requirements on you as a practitioner
- Expectations from associations/accreditation bodies/licence boards. This includes keeping data in line with the period of time a complaint can be raised against a professional under professional conduct procedures (BACP, n.d.)
- Data for client safeguarding, including where confidentiality needs to be breached to help the client where they reveal they may harm themselves
- Data for safeguarding others, including where confidentiality needs to be breached where a client indicates that they may harm others or are harming others
- Data for judicial purposes, for example, for court cases
- Requirements from insurers to retain data, in case of any eventual claim against your practice

Keeping proficient, clear, accurate records is of benefit to the practitioner as well as the client. Not having them can harm yourself as well as mean that you are not able to provide the best service possible to your client.

Data storage

In the previous chapters we looked at the vulnerability of data to cyberattacks. This included looking at the following:

Data being lost/altered
Data being exposed

Lost/altered data can impact a practitioner as follows:

1. They will be unable to fulfil requirements to hold client data for all the purposes noted in the previous section
2. Their business continuity/services to clients may be affected

Most readers will be aware of the importance of backing up data and not just having one copy kept statically on a single device. In the event something is deleted by accident or a device needs to be reinstalled or stops working, a backup copy can be used. Backup copies are similarly useful when data is lost, altered, or deleted due to a cyber incident.

Before we look at some guidance regarding storage options, let's look at a short conundrum faced by a therapist of many years – Joan.

Joan's conundrum

Can you store copies of client data on an external hard drive?

Joan has worked with clients for 30 years; she originally used notebooks to make her notes but has, for some time, used a computer. Her son, Max, turned up one day to visit with an external hard drive. He explained he had recently realised that he had deleted some important information that he didn't mean to. A clean-up he had done on his computer four months prior had been too thorough, something he didn't notice unfortunately until the deleted files had also long left the recycle bin of his cloud storage. Following advice from a friend, he was now backing up his data to an external drive. Knowing his mother wrote notes on all her clients, he suggested she consider doing the same.

Joan related to her son's story immediately. She recalled a time when she had just started working as a therapist and had by mistake thrown out a notebook she made notes of sessions in, when doing the cleaning. It had disrupted continuity in her practice as she was not able to look back on what her clients had said last. Joan also reflected on her obligations to keep records for a period of time.

Max showed her how she could make a copy to an external hard drive, say, once a month; then, she would have a relatively recent second copy if her computer went down.

The thing is, Joan feels uncertain about whether she is allowed to do this. She recently attended talks by her accreditation body on the GDPR rules, where practitioners were reminded to store sensitive data securely. She wonders if the external drive is secure, and what if she throws it out by mistake when cleaning as she had done with her notebook all those years before?

Activity

Before reading further, reflect on whether Joan can store client data on an external hard drive.

Joan's solution

As you may have seen through the different case studies, there are often some different thoughts that go into decisions when applying cybersecurity.

What Joan or someone in Joan's situation should do can be reflected on by revisiting the guiding stars of legislative requirements around data security/privacy for your location, expectations of accreditation bodies and also the cyber-risk of the storage point.

First, Joan might check the legislation and guidelines she adheres to for her practice. If there is nothing specific on where data can be stored, meaning nothing specific on the type of device, drive or other, then Joan might consider reviewing whether there is information on how confidential client records should be kept (format, duration). This will provide information towards what is permitted.

Finally, the cybersecurity view towards answering this is actually quite simple. The bottom line is that anyone holding confidential client records and wanting those records to be secure and safe should act as follows:

- They should operate a cybersecure practice
- They should back up important data
- They should store data securely, including protecting and encoding any client-sensitive information in a way that client data is as safe as possible. Thus, data needs to be stored in a way that it would be very difficult for anyone to access it, and for someone with unauthorised access to it, to work out who the data refers to

Through this book, we have covered a number of ways to secure devices. From that, the possible layers of security around any external hard drive,or external solid state drive (SSD), could be evaluated as follows:

- How is the external drive stored physically?
- Is the external drive password protected?
- Does the practitioner know where the external drive is at all times?
- Does only the practitioner have access to it, or do others as well?
- Is the data stored on it secured through the use of passwords, anonymisation, other?

Joan's decision

After finding there is nothing in the guidelines or legislation that she would be contravening, Joan decides to use the external device. Upon asking some peers, she finds out that some use external drives, while others use cloud storage. Joan, however, likes the idea of a physical copy on the small hard drive. It reminds her of her notebooks from before. Her son helps her install a password on it for opening it. They also together find a small fireproof lock box to put it in. Although she lives alone, Joan feels this is a good solution for her as through forming a habit to always take it out and put it back in the lock box it will be harder for her to lose it Joan also changes her way of storing client data to be fully anonymised and keeps a list of the anonymised names separately and in a way that it would be difficult for anyone to work out who her clients actually are.

Cloud storage

It is possible today to store files remotely on the servers of a cloud storage service provider. OneDrive, Dropbox and Google Drive are examples of well-known cloud storage providers. Cloud storage is another back up option to evaluate.

Many cloud storage solutions allow a user to keep a version of a document on their own device, and replicate a copy to cloud storage. Alternatively, documents may be kept just in the cloud storage and accessed from the device via the internet, as needed. With the first option, the document is then stored and kept on your computer, so it can be updated on the device when offline, and replicates to the cloud when online. With the latter option, where you store only on the cloud, access may be restricted when you are offline.

Do ensure to review any relevant legislation you are obliged to follow as to any restrictions on how you store data. Researchers, educators and practitioners working for companies with strict policies on where they store data should also check and apply the relevant policies when it comes to data storage. If this applies to you, check whether your workplace asks you to store on a cloud service and whether you are permitted to allow replication to your device.

From a practical point of view, most people will prefer to have their documents on their device and replicated to the cloud, as this can be more convenient for daily use. It also provides the practitioner with a backup copy. Thinking back to some of the cyberthreats mentioned earlier in the book, you may recall that malware leads to a compromised computer, where some form of software is installed that will cause harm and potentially data loss. Following such an attack, a device would first need to be fully cleaned and reinstalled by a professional. After that, provided the infection on the computer did not impact any files on a cloud service, the user can then redownload their files.

It is vital to remember is not to make the mistake of starting again with the same cybersecurity in place as before – with no improvements. Many companies have done this and found themselves quickly attacked again (Palmer, 2021). If you are ever victim of a cyber attack, ensure to revisit the chapters of this book to evaluate where to implement improvements and take advice from the professional helping you clean your device.

Cloud services themselves can be breached or hacked (Morag, 2021). If the malware that attacks your device or systems is sophisticated enough, it will also find your cloud storage. So, having only a cloud backup means that the practitioner is still vulnerable to data loss. Keeping other backups – for example, on a secure external drive, as in Joan's case – is one way to be prepared for any such wider attack. Many companies keep offline copies of data as a strategy in case they become victim to a ransomware attack.

The next section will provide tips when considering an external backup solution (on an external drive), but first some points that may guide you on how to select a cloud services provider to effectively and securely store client (or other) data:

- Some cloud storage providers have extra "security vault" folders with MFA logins to open them. If your cloud service offers this, this is where any client-sensitive data could be stored. Note, however, that threat actors will be very interested in what is in such a folder if your cloud storage is compromised. So, you might still consider splitting your client data up so that it is not all gathered there conveniently for them. If you ever get a 2FA/MFA alert from your cloud storage provider (or anything for that matter!) that is not generated by you, do not approve it, and take action to secure your first-level password immediately

- There are multiple resources online on which cloud storage providers are most secure in the present moment. Similar to the previous searches you have performed, look for "most secure cloud storage", and filter to the latest results. As you would have noted from earlier searches, many reviews are written in a way that anyone can understand them and, similarly here, you will not need technical knowledge to follow write ups on which cloud services provider has been breached the most and whether their features are up to date (Walker, 2021)
- One option to consider is replicating different folders to different cloud storages. Depending on how you log and separate client names and records, this may be another way to make it harder for someone with access to your records to connect them together

External storage

As in the conundrum with Joan, where legislation allows, practitioners can consider making periodic backups of files to a secure external drive. This means you have an offline copy of your files if something happens with your computer and cloud service storage.

Tips to consider:

- Buy an external drive that offers extra security, such as a password lock to open. Note that some external drives also offer a number of security features today, including remote erasure. As you have learnt earlier in the book, consider to research: "most secure external SSD/hard drive" – adding the relevant year to your search
- Place a reminder on your calendar to back up your files periodically
- Ensure a safe, secure storage place. Consider a lockable fire-proof box or safe so that you can still keep it relatively near your office/working space. This has a secondary benefit that, in the event of a fire, it may be a source of any lost files. It might be tempting to keep it far away from the original device with data on it; however, this may mean you lose sight of it. Also, having it too far away or in an inconvenient place means that it will not be easily accessible or retrievable when you need to back up your files. It does not take long to make a copy of files to an external drive, but it does take discipline to stay on schedule

Frequency of backups

This is tricky and can only be answered by yourself:

- If you do replicate your files to cloud storage, you might consider backing up data less frequently than if you don't. However, keep in mind the cyberattacks that can infiltrate cloud records

- Evaluate how far back on the calendar you could lose the latest records you have made but remember enough that you could replicate them
- Much also depends on the discipline of each person – most important is creating a good habit of making backups – so find a frequency where it does not feel like friction but rather like a simple, periodic task

Another benefit of backing up files to an external drive is that if you delete something you did not mean to (or change your mind), you may have a copy. Even if it is gone from your PC recycle bin, you may have it on your external drive. If you replicate to cloud storage, it might also still be there in the recycle bin, but note that cloud storage recycle bins are usually purged after a set period of time.

First steps after data exposure

For this, you do need to revert again to legislation and regulations relevant for your location and profession. The following, however, may provide some first steps and ideas from a security and cyber view, in conjunction with the tips already provided on what to do after a cyber incident:

- In the event of data exposure due to a cyberattack, a trained security professional can help you determine more precisely what has happened and give guidance on sanitation of your device, how far any infection may have gone and what has been affected. If you have been exposed to malware, they should be able to tell you which type – information that you can later use in any reporting. Knowing the type can also give an indication of how serious the problem may be, as some types are more commonplace and perhaps more is known about them, while others, run by the more professional criminal groups, may be more difficult to resolve
- You may also wish to contact any accreditation/licencing body you are affiliated with for advice on what to do if you have experienced a breach of your client data or to confirm any reporting actions they require of you
- If you are a researcher, your first point of reference may be a call to your ethics board for guidance. You will also need to ensure any breach is duly reported, as required by legislation in your location

On the victim side

After the breach in the Therapy centres in Finland in 2020, a volunteer organisation of Finnish cyber experts issued a very detailed checklist for victims of data breaches (KyberVPK – Community Cyber Response Force, 2020). A copy in English is available. Find the checklist by searching online for "Kyber VPK checklist for victims of a data breach".

Some of the points are a valuable guideline for anyone who has similarly been a victim of a breach of sensitive data. It can also be worth taking two minutes to read through it yourself to get an idea of the impact a data breach can have on one of your clients and why the journey through this book has been worth it.

Remember, before you ever send such a list to a client, that the legislation of your country is your first obligation. If that legislation includes information on how to inform your clients, that is what you should follow first and foremost.

Summary

Keeping client data safe (particularly when working within a health-sector-related profession, where data is valuable to criminals) needs more than ticking legislative boxes or saying practitioners store data securely. It needs practitioners to *actually* keep data securely and ensure the privacy of their clients operationally (Lustgarten et al., 2020).

While legislation around data protection and privacy has helped bring to the fore these important topics, as of the time of writing, there remains scant texts regarding expectations on cybersecurity and little guidance on how to actually achieve data security in most ethics codes or guidelines for practitioners.

Among other topics, this chapter has covered the following:

- Clarified the importance of a layered approach to cybersecurity in order to secure client data
- Provided deeper understanding of why practitioners must only use secure networks, implement security software on devices and verify the security standards and capabilities of all products used, including online communications tools
- Unpacked the importance of knowing all the data sets a practitioner holds about their clients and the potential consequences of exposure of any form of client data
- Clarified potential ways to store, handle and eventually delete data – including an explanation of why deletion on a timely basis is important
- Enabled deeper insights into the rationale behind legislation and regulation around data protection and privacy, along with a reminder that legislation exists to ensure privacy and data protection for all of us
- Provided tips on being transparent with clients on cyber-risks around their data and informing them in a positive, proactive way
- Clarified from a cybersecurity perspective some of the first steps to take in the event of a data breach

Ethics and data have been at the heart of each chapter so far; this chapter has just enabled more insight into the inextricable link between cybersecurity, data security and ethics. Cybersecurity helps practitioners make choices to actually achieve data security, which underlies the ethics and confidentiality expectations around their professions.

References

American Counseling Association. (2014). *ACA code of ethics*. https://www.counseling .org/knowledge-center/ethics

British Association for Counselling and Psychotherapy. (2018). *Ethical framework for the counselling professions*. https://www.bacp.co.uk/events-and-resources/ethics-and-standards/ethical-framework-for-the-counselling-professions/

British Association for Counselling and Psychotherapy. (2020, March 6). *Government update on statutory regulation of counsellors and psychotherapists*. https://www .bacp.co.uk/news/news-from-bacp/2020/6-march-government-update-on-statutory-regulation-of-counsellors-and-psychotherapists/

British Association for Counselling and Psychotherapy. (n.d.). *FAQs about GDPR: A quick guide to the new general data protection regulation*. https://www.bacp.co.uk/about-us /contact-us/gdpr/

The British Psychological Society. (2018). *The general data protection regulation (GDPR) – FAQs*. https://www.bps.org.uk/news-and-policy/general-data-protection-regulation-gdpr-%E2%80%93-faqs

European Association of Psychotherapy. (2018). *EAP statement of ethical principles*. https:// www.europsyche.org/quality-standards/eap-guidelines/statement-of-ethical-principles/

Global Code of Ethics. (2021). https://www.globalcodeofethics.org/

Information Commissioner's Office. (n.d.). *Guide to the UK general data protection regulation (UK GDPR)*. Crown Copyright. https://ico.org.uk/for-organisations/guide-to-data-protection/guide-to-the-general-data-protection-regulation-gdpr/

International Coaching Federation. (2019). *Updated ICF core competencies*. https://coach-ingfederation.org/core-competencies

Griffiths, K. E., & Campbell, M. A. (2008). Regulating the regulators: Paving the way for international, evidence-based coaching standards. *International Journal of Evidence Based Coaching and Mentoring, 6*(1), 19–31. https://radar.brookes.ac.uk/radar /file/8cc34160-8136-4dd2-b185-1cdd24c6984f/1/vol06issue1-paper-02.pdf

Hirani, K. (2017). Transcending ethical dilemmas in coaching and supervision: A model to develop a transpersonal perspective. *Philosophy of Coaching: An International Journal, 2*(1), 6–27. http://doi.org/10.22316/poc/02.1.02

Ivtzan, I., & Lomas, T. (2016). *Mindfulness in positive psychology: The science of meditation and wellbeing*. London: Routledge.

KyberVPK – Community Cyber Response Force. (2020). *Checklist for victims of a data breach*. https://kybervpk.fi/en/releases/checklist-for-victims-of-a-data-breach/

Lorenzen, M. (2022, January 7). *It-leverandør til danske læger ramt af ransomware: Sådan afværgede de katastrofen*. Version 2. https://www.version2.dk/artikel/it-leverandoer-danske-laeger-ramt-ransomware-saadan-afvaergede-de-katastrofen-1093960

Lustgarten, S. D., Garrison, Y. L., Sinnard, M. T., & Flynn, A. W. (2020). Digital privacy in mental healthcare: Current issues and recommendations for technology use. *Current Opinion in Psychology, 36*, 25–31. https://doi.org/10.1016/j.copsyc.2020.03.012

Morag, S. (2021, December 15). *Why cloud storage isn't immune to ransomware*. Dark Reading. https://www.darkreading.com/attacks-breaches/why-cloud-storage-isn-t-immune-to-ransomware

Palmer, D. (2021, April 5). *Ransomware: A company paid millions to get their data back but forgot to do one thing. So, the hackers came back again.* ZDNet. https://www.zdnet.com/article/ransomware-this-is-the-first-thing-you-should-think-about-if-you-fall-victim-to-an-attack/

Shackelford, S. J. (2019). Should cybersecurity be a human right? Exploring the "shared responsibility" of cyber peace (2017). *Stanford Journal of International Law No. 2019, Kelley School of Business Research Paper No. 17–55.* http://doi.org/10.2139/ssrn.3005062

Stopforth, M. (2019). Establishing training routes in coaching psychology. *Coaching Psychologist, 15*(1), 76–77. https://shop.bps.org.uk/the-coaching-psychologist-vol-15-no-1-june-2019

Walker, D. (2021, April 13). *Cloud storage: How secure are Dropbox, OneDrive, Google Drive, and iCloud?* ITPro. https://www.itpro.co.uk/cloud-security/34663/cloud-storage-how-secure-are-dropbox-onedrive-google-drive-and-icloud

Chapter 9

Case studies

Introduction

Do wait to read these case studies in line with being pointed to them in different chapters. Try not to read them ahead of that, and do not be tempted to read them altogether if you come across them in skimming through the book after purchase.

They are purposefully built to provide an opportunity to start to use the knowledge in the book and train picking up on what is happening in the different scenarios yourself. Of course, after reading the book, you can return to repeat a read through of all of them and see if you read them differently a second time around.

Each case study is written as a story around one person, providing information on what has happened and giving moments for pause to reflect. Reading through, reflections should start to come up, and you are encouraged to write them down as they do. Later, you can go through your notes and evaluate how you are starting to spot red flags and see cybersecurity in a contextual sense.

The reason the case studies are referred to in the chapters of the book is that they are put in as optional/extra reading at the time of a chapter that has similar content, or to prepare you for upcoming material. The case studies also are progressively a little more difficult, starting at Level 1 and going through to Level 3. Again, you will get more out of them by waiting for the relevant reference point to read them, and not getting ahead of that.

Note there are different possible reasons the attacks in the three case studies occur and the outcomes given are one of those options. Where you come up with other thoughts and explanations as you read, this is good; do not see it as you have answered incorrectly. It shows you are starting to see the various ways the cyberspace can be exploited.

The elements and the events depicted in each case study are based on real-life cybercrime and fraud scenarios. However, the compilation of the events, the story telling and the names in the case studies are fictional.

DOI: 10.4324/9781003184805-10

The full case of Adrian (Level 1)

I became really frustrated by it all. I realise it was my own lack of knowledge, but it would be easier if cybercrime didn't exist, and I didn't have to think about these things.

Adrian

This story is divided into two parts, so you get to pause and start to form your own thoughts before getting more information. Adrian's story highlights how having a little knowledge about security can easily stop much cybercrime pretty quickly. So, absorbing the information and tips in this book can go a long way in securing your practice.

Let's meet Adrian

- Adrian has been coaching for most of his life. It is simply everything to him
- He does most of his work face to face, but also uses an online video conferencing product with some clients who want to work with him but live too far to travel. He has always used the same product. If you asked him before the cyberattack, he would proudly say he was one of the first users of the software and he knows everything about it. If you ask him now, you will hear him grumble a little and change the subject. This whole experience he describes as disruptive and frustrating

Part 1

In January, Adrian woke up to find he couldn't post on a social media site as he sometimes does. Everything was closed, even worse, not only his personal page was closed down but also a company page he had linked to it and was administrator of.

It didn't take too long to find out what had happened. Some of his friends had emailed him to warn that it looked like his page had been hacked. When Adrian appealed to the site to reopen everything, they refused, explaining that hackers had put content on the pages that was a breach of the social media site's rules. Adrian relented and opened a new private page and company page and carried on, putting it all behind him.

In February, Adrian's friends called him: why was he sending them emails with invoices asking them for payment? He had no idea. After receiving a couple of these back from them he realised his email had been hacked. Luckily, it wasn't the email he used with his clients, so none of them had received anything. Adrian took this as meaning little damage had been done. He updated the password on his private email account and put it all behind him.

In March, Adrian was on an online conferencing tool with a client. Halfway through the session, his computer started working really slowly but they managed to complete the session.

Activity

Open your reflective notes:

1. What have you picked up from the story so far?
2. What do you think Adrian should be concerned about at this stage?
3. What do you think will happen next for Adrian, or how this will conclude?

Take a break of at least five to ten minutes before moving to Part 2

Part 2

After your break, open your reflective notes again.

Add any new thoughts to what you might be concerned about if you were in Adrian's position and what you think could happen next.

When you are ready, read on.

After talking to his client online, Adrian finished his day. The next morning, he found an email from someone saying they had hacked his computer and quoting some sentences from the coaching call where his computer had started working slowly. He would not have believed it, except that he remembered the words as clearly as they were written in the email.

Panicking slightly, he rang a friend and they talked it through. His friend agreed, it sounded really strange but there had been a lot of media reports lately on how easy it was to hack the software Adrian was using. Not sure what to do, Adrian decided to take his computer to a security professional. After explaining his client call and story, Adrian added in that he was just tired of all these strange things: first his social media pages, then his email, now this. The security professional looked at him and asked him to give more information on the other events.

After Adrian finished going through it all, the security professional asked Adrian if he had different passwords on all those accounts. Adrian was getting tired of all the explaining by now. Flustered, he explained that he had an extremely secure password with numbers, symbols and all kinds of elements. More than enough, and he used it consistently everywhere.

The security professional went to work and called Adrian back in later. He explained he hadn't found any malware on this computer but recommended that he cleaned it and reset it. He then informed Adrian that he thought his password had been leaked and was likely up for sale on the darknet or otherwise in the hands of criminals. He explained that using the same password consistently everywhere is the wrong approach; instead, there should be no repetition. The security professional brought up that Adrian is very well known and visible on the internet and perhaps had been persistently targeted by fraudsters seeking some good information on any important, well-known clients that he might have. He also explained to Adrian that he was lucky as none of the criminals who used his password on his social media site, email or the conferencing tool appeared very sophisticated. Furthermore, there was nothing to indicate they had hacked into more than that one call – as they had acted quickly afterwards, revealing themselves. More sophisticated fraudsters might have waited and attended more calls over time.

Adrian went home and followed instructions to change all his passwords, and make them unique per login, using another device while his computer was cleaned. He reported a data breach to the relevant authorities where he lived – on the intercepted call and had an honest discussion with his client about it and informed them how this would not happen again. His client wasn't very happy but decided to continue to work with him. Adrian also installed MFA wherever he was able. He has, so far, not had any new problems.

Activity

Open your reflective notes:

1. Note what comes up for you when you read this case – in terms of feelings, reactions or observations
2. What have you actioned so far that will prevent you from being like Adrian?
3. Rate on a scale of 1–10, where 10 is high, how effectively you analysed this case study section by section

Your answers as to what happened in the case study are less important than how you analysed the sections and what your thought processes were. What happened to Adrian could have also come from malware, which many of you will have noted as the cause. The different layers of how the criminal used Adrian's password were there to encourage good reflexivity as you read bit by bit. Adrian was fortunate, as a more sophisticated criminal would have moved to a more extensive attack.

Challenges and observations

- Facing an incident like this was difficult for Adrian as it was disruptive over some months
- He describes the security aspects of his new set-up, after the cyberattack, with multiple complex passwords and MFA as "frustrating", which is very understandable. He misses the simplicity of using the same password for everything
- It will be important that Adrian doesn't just push the event into the past and forget about it. Instead, he needs to turn it around for some motivation to propel himself into action to continuously secure his practice against cybersecurity issues. If fraudsters found him an easy target this time, they might try again
- Adrian was unaware of the vulnerability in using the same password everywhere, no matter how "strong" it was. So, it is likely there are other areas of the cybersecurity of his practice that could be improved upon

You can now return to reading the book and building your skills towards not ending up like Adrian.

*

The full case of Perky (Level 2)

I realised afterwards, putting myself in the clients' shoes, that even if the criminal never figured out my clients' names, there was still this sense of exposure and breach of the client confidentiality I promise them when we talk.

Perky

Perky's story will allow you to check your reflective thinking and activate some of your learning so far. As you read each section, enable your own thoughts to come forward, write them in your reflective notes, pause to think a bit deeper and then move to the next part and so forth.

Let's meet Perky

- Perky is a leading counselling professor who has spent some years working at a top university in France. He spends vacation times and the summer every year at his flat in New York, where he reconnects face-to-face with some of his clients there. Perky has a number of qualifications and prides himself on his client base. He also travels extensively to attend conferences and to deliver lectures
- His services to private clients include an extensive package, aimed at helping top professionals balance the issues they come to him about, alongside working high-powered jobs in New York. He offers follow-ups online when he is not in town
- Perky has worked like this for the last 5 years. Over time, he has become more efficient, being able to keep up with clients when they need him, even from airports, hotels and on the move. He has never found it hard to log-on from networks wherever he is, enabling him to keep earning a high income and his client base on track

Part 1

Let's get straight to it: Perky has fallen victim to a ransomware attack. He has received a message asking him to buy Bitcoins equivalent to US$50,000 to regain access to his computer and files. Perky is determined not to pay but is in a dilemma because a security professional has said that his computer will need to be fully cleaned and he has no backup of the files that are now locked up on there. He had a few things on cloud storage, but they too have been hacked.

To make matters worse, the ransomers have made it clear that if he does not pay, they intend to sell copies of his client documents on the darknet. Perky is not only aware of which of his well-established clients would quickly make the news if his notes on them got out, he is also aware that he has not, at all times, anonymised their names. The ransomers have also sent proof that they have his data and are aware of the names of the clients the press would be interested in. They have sent him copies of his non-high-profile clients' information as well. As he works with clients who have some very sensitive issues, Perky is extremely concerned.

Passive-to-active

- While Perky had noticed his computer had been slower for some weeks, he had not paid attention that this might be a red flag. Often, ransomware is deployed sometime after malware has been downloaded. In that period, the computer may work abnormally, and the criminals take their time to look and find documents before making themselves visible, starting the ransomware attack and locking the computer or encrypting the files
- One day, Perky turned on his computer and could only watch as all the icons on his desktop – of which he had quite a few – started to turn into what looked like pieces of paper. At that time, he thought it was updating, but then came up a message on the screen from the attackers informing him of their demands
- Perky has been through the mandatory cybersecurity training at the university, but has not really paid attention to it and has never looked at the security of his computer
- One good thing is that the malware has not further infiltrated the university. This is because the attack occurred on a private laptop that Perky used separately with his private clients, as it was lighter to travel with and easier to connect to a network wherever he was on the road

Activity

Open your reflective notes:

1. What do you note as alarming so far in the case?
2. Where do you think Perky's computer was compromised?
3. Based on what you have learnt so far, what do you think Perky has done wrong?

Take a break of at least five to ten minutes before moving to Part 2.

Part 2

There are countless ways malware can get onto a computer – through websites, links, files, apps and other. You may have noticed Perky spent a lot of time on the road, calling clients from airports, hotels and conference centres all over the world. Perky was glad to see Wi-Fi wherever he was and to connect to it (particularly if it was free). He had no understanding of the cyber risks associated with public Wi-Fi.

- Perky talked extensively to the security professional he hired to help him after the ransomware attack. He learned there was no guarantee that the threat actors would honour their word, release his documents back to him, and not publish them if he paid a ransom. He also understood the ethical dilemma of paying up. In the end, however, he decided to pay the ransom
- Once he paid, Perky was given his files back, and the security professional fully sanitised the computer as well as found an expert who checked the darknet to see if anything had been leaked. So far, they haven't found anything but have promised to help Perky with how to deal with this if something is published later. (Note to reader: please remember this is a fictional case study and that Perky was lucky!) Current statistics show double extortion is increasing, with threat actors still selling data even if they receive a ransom and that not all victims are able to fully restore their data after a ransom is paid (ENISA, 2020; Muhammad, 2021)
- Determined that this should never happen again, Perky has revised how he stores documents
- Perky took the weeks after the incident very hard, becoming anxious about what could happen to his clients, although the data had not been released. Guilt also came up for him: first, that he had not really fulfilled ethical requirements on his side to keep what his clients shared with him safe, and second, that he had paid criminals a sum of money. Not being able to stop thinking about everything, Perky realised he was experiencing the aftermath of being a cybercrime victim and signed up for some therapy sessions for himself
- After working through his emotions, he ended up destroying the laptop that was breached. He bought a new one, to give himself a sense of starting over. He put it on a security software suite that he had researched thoroughly. He also added an extra malware detection program that he runs like clockwork
- Some months on, Perky has bounced back. He no longer talks to clients over public Wi-Fi when he travels; instead, he has extended his mobile phone coverage so he can hotspot from that. It has increased his mobile phone bills when he is travelling, but he now sees that as being what he has to pay for wanting to keep on working when on the road

- After finding stories online about some ransomers demanding increased payments or still publishing the materials after they get the ransom, Perky does actually feel lucky, particularly because he has also seen the sums of money hackers sometimes ask for. Since some of his clients were very well known, if the hackers had revealed his documents, his practice might have been ruined
- He has been open with people around him about what happened, even providing some training to staff in his department at the university so that they might avoid having the same happen to them. He makes sure they know that this is not just about preventing a hacker but about fulfilling promises – saying: we promise that our work with clients is confidential and that is how it should be. He expresses often when he talks how he imagines himself in the shoes of a client and how he would feel if information about him was exposed
- He reported the breach to the data authorities in the countries where he operates

---

Activity

Open your reflective notes:

1. Reflect on how you analysed this case study through the sections. Have you started to pick up on red flags or other factors any differently than before reading the chapters you have read so far?
2. If you have any behaviours or practices similar to Perky, what will you change going forward?
3. If you have not been putting into action the steps indicated in this book so far, reflect on whether you need to go back and find the action points and think again
4. Rate on a scale of 1–10, where 10 is high, how effectively you analysed this case study section by section

---

Challenges and observations

Note that Perky's case was a ransomware case. This involved blackmail and a situation where his documents were locked and unavailable for use. This meant his business was also fully offline for the period of time he was resolving what to do.

You can now return to reading the book and building skills towards not ending up like Perky.

*

The full case of Delores (Level 3)

> It's been important for me to be open with my clients that this hap-
> pened. I didn't know any better then, but I sure do now. Trust me, now
> I tell them how good I am at protecting their data today, and I mean
> actually, really trying to protect it. I also ensure they know their part
> in ensuring all our interactions together are as safe as possible.
>
> *Delores*

Delores' story will allow you to check your detective skills. As you
read each section, enable your own questions to come forward, note
them in your reflective notes, pause to think a bit deeper, then move
to the next part and so forth. Delores hopes her story will provide
learning for others.

Let's meet Delores

- Delores has been building her business for some time; she is
  determined to make it big as a coach. She decided early on in her
  career that her niche is working online and always being ready to
  go the extra mile with availability for her clients
- Delores offers packages where her clients get an hour of coaching,
  can write three emails to her between appointments and chat via
  SMS when they need her extra support. Clients who don't want
  the extra support can also just take coaching sessions with her
- All her work with clients is carefully contracted, so that both
  sides are clear on how they want to work together
- After working like this for three years, she has become very used
  to it and her business runs like clockwork

Part 1

Delores has just reported a data breach. She has been blackmailed by
a criminal who has gained access to her mobile phone. After receiving
screenshots of some of her SMS conversations via mobile phone apps,
she realised this was serious. The criminal has made it clear that they
have figured out who the clients are by tracing the mobile numbers on
public directories. Also, that they are going to reveal all the information
if she does not pay them.

Challenges

- This is a case where someone has gained unauthorised access to Delores' device through malware and are targeting the data they can get most value for
- Unfortunately, Delores did not think about stopping to use her phone initially, giving the criminal more data
- One good thing is that Delores always contracted to converse with her clients via mobile apps. Only clients who wanted this part of the service have potentially been exposed; however, on the other hand, Delores had never made the risks of using apps clear to them. Additionally, she never security checked the apps she uses and always just said yes to whichever app the client wanted to use

Activity

Open your reflective notes:

1. What do you think Delores should do now to protect her practice better in the future?
2. Should she still use apps, going forward, when this is all sorted out? If so, what else does she need to put in place regarding security and informing her clients

Take a break of at least five to ten minutes before moving to Part 2

Part 2

- Delores contacted a security professional, who disabled her phone fully from the internet. Delores then wrote down the names of all the clients who had conversations ongoing with her on the apps that were hacked. The professional then fully cleaned the device
- Delores also started to dig into what happened herself. Researching the name the blackmailer is using online, she has found out that they are likely to just keep asking for more money even if she did pay
- The criminal indicated that they had files of five clients across two apps. They did not appear to have accessed any of the other apps and conversations
- Delores contacted the impacted clients. Most of them were newer clients and had not shared so much with her. She then contacted all of the clients she

worked with over apps that were not exposed and explained the situation. She informed them that her support to them over chat would resume after she had researched an app she felt secure about and after their next 1:1 sessions with her, when they could re-contract on: the risks, what should and should not be sent over chat and deletion
- Despite this being a difficult time, Delores kept calm once she realised what was happening, reporting the data breach and making a detailed report with law enforcement

---

Activity

Open your reflective notes:

1. What is commendable about Delores' response?
2. How do you think you would react if something happened?

Conclusions

- Despite initially not grasping that she was experiencing a cyberattack and still using a compromised device, in the end Delores actually reacted really well. She remained level-headed, researched the situation and made clear decisions. By reporting the data breach and being honest with her clients, she also handled this appropriately
- Her business was down for a while, when she had to close everything to find out what was happening, and this has cost her some earnings. At the same time, this was the right thing to do. It might also help repair any damage to her reputation, as she took time to resolve and come back more secure
- Through reading around what happened to her, Delores now knows it would be advisable to take all devices fully offline during such an attack. Next time, she knows she would also react quicker to an incident

---

Activity

Open your reflective notes:

1. Evaluate how you formed thoughts as you went through the different sections of this case study
2. Have you started to think how you would respond to a cyber event yourself?

3. Reflect on how, once you have some knowledge about security, it is easier to consider how to make it more secure
4. Rate on a scale of 1–10, where 10 is high, how effectively you analysed this case study section by section.
5. Review all your ratings through the three case studies and note where you have improved

You can now return to reading the book and building skills towards not ending up like Delores.

*

Chapter 10

Checklists and conclusions

Armed and ready

The journey through this book has been through concrete examples, alongside practical, active application and analytical, abstract and reflective thinking. Some readers may have noted that this at points matches elements of Kolb's (1984) experiential learning theory. This has been intentional, so as to equip you to continue alone, along with your new toolkit.

Before reviewing all your new resources, let's take a moment to acknowledge that this book will have opened your eyes in many ways. In some of the chapters you were encouraged to positively view the sense of work that comes with cybersecurity, the friction of extra controls/defence layers and the at times frightening statistics. This is perhaps a trick from coaching psychology, to set a new view, but it is the case that anything concerning, alarming or – let's be frank and use the word again – frightening – will stay that way if we are not aware of it and don't do something about it. Without the friction and hard work you would not now be more secure.

If you had not read this book, you would still be operating professionally within a realm of not knowing the threats around you and how to set up your practice to be more secure against them. As has been noted, it is often the human who is cited as the weak link in a cybersecurity set-up (Wiederhold, 2014). Awareness is key.

As you move into operating alone, the different activities in each section can be revisited any time you need to refresh. The checklists through the book, and the extra ones at the end, you can bookmark and use (and even adapt) as needed. If something ever happens, some of the checklists may serve as a companion to you in the early steps of determining how to resolve a cyber incident and then recover from it. In essence, you are no longer alone in this.

Even as you were reading chapters, perhaps media stories around security and fraud started to stand out in a new way. Continue to explore, and next time do read everything in a security alert from authorities or the bank. Relate it to your learning in these chapters and continue to reflect on how a) you would respond yourself and b) evaluate if and how your practice is secure from the threat.

DOI: 10.4324/9781003184805-11

Healthcare, as an industry, will continue to be attacked regularly, and the threats specified in this book will continue to exist. Cybersecurity's future is bright, however, with children who are coming into a technology-reliant world now being informed on cybersecurity from a young age (Barefoot Computing, n.d.) and university courses on the subject flourishing. Governments are also finally turning towards how they will combat the large crime rings executing malware and ransomware attacks (Ransomware Task Force, 2021) and even starting to talk together at, for example, the G7 level on tackling the problem together (Palmer, 2021).

Any impact from these positive initiatives will though take considerable time to be seen. Therefore, it is the author's opinion that, in the coming years, the emphasis within cybersecurity should continue to be on building up what people and businesses can do for themselves. It is also the author's opinion that more companies will start to say no to paying ransom demands to cybercriminals and continue to internally equip themselves better. Alongside building defences, companies may also investigate and implement smarter ways to store backup data and find new, adaptive ways to make data difficult to interpret and resell once outside of company walls.

This evolution will take time, but you have now joined the ranks of a cyber-informed professional performing precisely those steps. You have, through the action points, layered your defences, looked at how you secure and back up your data, as well as started to learn your role in spotting red flags and abnormalities to ensure that you are also an active, strong part of your cybersecurity set-up.

Now to the promised review of your new toolkit. There is a lot that can be listed, but some of the main overarching abilities gained through this book can be condensed as follows:

- Awareness about cyberthreats most applicable to your practice
- Competencies towards being able to detect and mitigate cyberattacks and attempted fraud
- Knowledge of some of the language and terminology used in cybersecurity
- New practices, procedures, behaviours and checks in place to keep your practice as secure as possible
- Skills towards spotting red flags and taking a pause to thoroughly check out any situation where there are abnormalities
- Realisation that it is not difficult to perform research on the security of the tools and products you use
- More conscious control over how safe your cyber environment is – compared with just applying some security or controls ad hoc
- Confidence to, going forward, read and absorb information on new threats in the cyberspace, aware that, very often, they are new combinations of existing threats
- Ongoing competences to maintain the enhanced security that has been implemented through the reflective activities and action points of this book

- Improved understanding of ethics and privacy and data laws from a new view of why they are in place and their connection to cybersecurity
- Ability to more competently mitigate the risk of any breaches of data or confidentiality from a practical, security point of view

Scenarios and situations not covered in this book may come up as you now continue on the path. If they do, stay calm at all times and recentre. Look again and connect aspects of what is coming up to something else you have learnt. Apply the foundations you now have in new ways. There can be a trend in the media to make anything look new and shiny, meaning that when reading about a "new" scam, look closely at all the elements to find out what is the actual story, and the media packaging. Often, it's an old scam with a new coat. Remember also that you will be reviewing and researching the security software tools you use now on a more regular basis. They will also evolve. So, while new cyberthreats will come to pass or existing ones change design or evolve, so will you – and your toolkit.

Cybercrime is a growing, fast-changing world, where criminals will always be trying to find ways through defences. Keep learning, your future research and choices will keep your practices and clients as safe as possible. Also, you have now implemented good, ethical standards around a number of important security topics, and can, going forward, consider yourself a more cybersecure practitioner.

Final reflections and actions

Just a couple of more tasks before the end of this journey:

1. As you look through the checklists coming up, bookmark any that will be useful ongoing to embed your learning into practice on your new pathway as a cybersecure practitioner
2. Open your reflective notes one final time

    - What did you write on the first page? How did you respond then about what you knew about cybersecurity, at the start of this journey?
    - Add today's date on a new page or under the original section. Add some notes on what you know about cybersecurity today
    - What are your top five learnings from this book?
    - What is the one particular thing that you have read that has stayed with you? Note how you could pass this on to another person this week – a peer practitioner, someone in your family or someone else that you know
    - What do you want to learn about next when it comes to cybersecurity?
    - Note any practical steps you still need to put into practice. Add deadlines for each to your calendar or diary

The author would welcome receiving some of your responses to these bullet points. If you feel like sharing, please send them (information on how to connect is in the afterword).

*

Checklists

Minimum steps when setting up a new device or computer

Take advice from an IT professional, as needed, in addition to following this checklist

☐	Add only to a secure network
☐	Ensure that firewall is enabled and security software is installed (including any updates)
☐	Download and install updates to operating system or firmware
☐	Ensure security software is set up
☐	Even if you have a brand new device, perform a full security scan before enabling any cloud service, software or moving files to the device
☐	Consult the user manual for the device, particularly if it is a new brand/model to you, look for information on any security features that it has
☐	Remove any software you do not need and will not use. Don't leave it "in case"; you can always reinstall it at a later date
☐	Change any default passwords that the device came with
☐	Enable secure locks on the device. Do not use an obvious pin and enable biometric locks where possible
☐	Only when all security steps are complete, including any other points you research for yourself, enable access to any documents or cloud storage or move files onto the device
☐	For second-hand devices, while the aforementioned steps can still be used, also research further on how to perform full and detailed sanitation of the device before you do anything else

Further guidance

Consult a government-linked website, for example, if you search "NCSC + securing devices" the results will return a page with useful tips. (NCSC, 2019).

*

Red flags checklist

The points here pull together some of the pointers in the book on spotting red flags. Add any others you have noted for yourself as important.

Summary version:

- Abnormal behaviour, demand or request
- Pushy language/time pressure (though take note that fraudsters today are aware this is a well-cited red flag and some can be extremely patient)
- Unusual payment methods suggested
- Something simply does not make sense
- Emotional conversation or content

More detail:

- Don't ignore red flags or that intuitive sense something is wrong
- The reason that banks are always telling you do not give out your login credentials (password, pin, MFA information) is that the only people that need those are you and criminals trying to steal from you! Your bank, someone from your bank, someone from the government, tax or other authority/business/other does not need your login credentials to look up your information and/or to help you. They just need to find you in their systems, often via a customer number or case number
- A genuine caller from an authority or bank will not push you or rush you. This is what criminals do, trying to catch you off guard to make a fast decision
- A genuine caller will not try to put you in a fear-based place or any other state to elicit a negative emotional response from you
- A properly trained employee will not be angry or frustrated if you have questions or inform them that you would like to check a couple of things, then call them back through the main office direct line
- Remember criminals can spoof phone numbers, the music in the background of a call, copy websites, SMS, emails and more. You are their business. Don't make them rich!

- Commit the internet search phrase "Is xyz a scam?" to memory. Making a quick search whether the story you have been told comes up as a scam might be the best internet search you can ever do

Do not ignore your instincts
If something sounds too good to be true – it probably is

*

Apps checklist

Take care to check apps before you download:

- ☑ Are they on a reputable app store?
- ☑ Are they commonly used?
- ☑ Do they have a good rating?
- ☑ Any red flags? If yes, perform more checks about the app
- ☑ Do you know anyone who uses it?
- ☑ When still in doubt, do not download!

*

Creating "stop-and-think" checklists

This book has focused on threats pertaining to your business. However, some of the defences you have put in place, along with the skills you have learnt, can transfer further.

This checklist you create yourself. The idea is to build a list of behaviours you need to be better at adopting or checks you want to be reminded to do across your business or private use of the cyberspace. Look through the reflective notes you kept during the chapters for inspiration of items you might want to add.

Example Version 1

Here are some example points to put in a "stop-and-think" checklist aimed at yourself. Make your own using your own points and style of wording:

- Did you expect what you are about to click on or open? If not, stop and think
- Are you about to download something you do not know the source of? If yes, why?
- I will stop to check my bank accounts on a frequent basis. I will think about how to set up a reminder to do this until it becomes automatic to me
- . . . . (add as many points as you want)
- . . . .

Example Version 2

If you have a family or other household members sharing your cyberspace, create a "stop-and-think" checklist to introduce cybersecurity to them as well. This will make your home network safer for all the devices on it. For content of the checklist, consider what each member of the household uses technology for and where the risks may be.

If you have younger children, use alternative language suitable for their age group. Try to make it fun where possible so that they are encouraged to follow it – for example, you could have a points-system where they are rewarded for applying the checklist items.

Here are some example points to put in a "stop-and-think" checklist aimed at a household with young children:

15 points – I will stop and check with my parents before I click to download any new games

50 points – I never reply to messages from people I know before showing them to my parents

The examples given are just to provide some starter inspiration. Write in a style that suits your household and use points that cover your needs. Remember if you put this in place, to always be supportive when a family member comes to check with you something on the list – you have put it there for a reason so spend time to review with them.

Consider also researching points related to keeping children safe online and incorporating these to your checklists. There are also a growing number of resources, such as the Barefoot Computing (n.d.) campaign, that can also be leveraged. Another consideration is to write a version for any vulnerable family members who need to take extra care of not being manipulated.

*

Data privacy reminders checklist

- Review your implementation of data privacy legislation for your location
- Review the guidelines issued by the accreditation bodies, associations or authorities you are a member of or licenced by
- Research other sources of information on data privacy relevant to your exact profession
- Ensure you have written information about cyber risks available for your clients (perhaps as part of any materials you provide during contracting)
- **Review** your data deletion practices

- Are your files set up in a way you can consistently delete them in line with requirements?
- Do you need to schedule a reminder to review which files to delete?
- Don't forget to delete all client related traces
- Never keep chat messages on tablet or phone devices longer than absolutely necessary; discourage your clients from using chat apps for sharing any confidential information
- Where still in doubt about anything, reach out to a legal professional

*

Credentials checklist

- Use strong passwords/passphrases
- Do not use the same password everywhere. You will now know why from the chapters of this book!
- Use 2FA or MFA where available. Never be frustrated with the friction; it is there to protect you. Remember some of the cases in this book and change your response
- If your password is compromised, always change any security questions you have logged
- Do not share passwords, 2FA/MFA codes or any other login credentials with anyone. Your credentials are your own. No matter what story you are told, remember that the only person that needs them really is you
- If you need help with your banking, arrange a power of attorney with your bank. Never give another party your own login, no matter how trusted they are to you
- If you write passwords/passphrases down, ensure to code them in a way no one can understand them or what they are for. Never add them to a document or notes file you create in your device; instead, consider using a trusted, thoroughly researched password manager as needed

*

Compromised email addresses checklist

Did you know you can see if your personal email address or phone number has been part of a data breach?

https://haveibeenpwned.com/

This is a website that was created by Troy Hunt in 2013. Thousands revert to it daily to check if their data has been part of a compromise. The same website has a checker for passwords that have been compromised in breaches and may therefore be more vulnerable going forward:

https://haveibeenpwned.com/Passwords

There are plans for the FBI to add compromised passwords into this database (Hunt, 2021).

Keep in mind this website can only provide an indication – it do not have all records of all possible breached email addresses/passwords.

Actions if your email address has been compromised:

Now that you have read this book, if you discover that your email has been compromised, you should feel competent and ready to take action. Start by researching the latest tips on what to do. For an email breach, the advice you will find may include the following: run a full virus scan, change your password, change your security questions, install MFA or 2FA and stay extra vigilant to any red flags immediately after the breach.

*

Recovery from a cyber incident or fraud

Some tips for when you have resolved an incident or fraud case:

Practice self-compassion. There is no silver bullet to preventing cyberattacks or fraud. Cybercriminals can be very prepared and operate very sophisticated attacks. If, at the time of the event, you were operating as securely as possible, revisit chapters in this book to rebuild your confidence. Recheck your cyber defences so that you recalibrate back in a place of knowing you are doing what you can.

If you were not operating as securely as you should have been, reread the book, follow the action points and check all your cyber defences.

Take advice, as needed, from professionals on where the weakness was and take steps to improve. Companies have been reattacked when they have not changed anything in their security after an attack, and threat actors tried again (Palmer, 2021).

Continue to monitor your bank accounts frequently and be vigilant to all transactions made. Do this especially in the period after the incident, but it is also a recommended regular practice for anyone.

Cybercrime and fraud victims each have painful stories to tell. Some need support after an incident to get back to feeling safe again. Ask for help if and when you need it. Check for fraud victim support groups in your location, or online.

*

Government level resources

The governments and authorities of most countries have great resources for fraud-related information. Look for them online for your country of residence. Take care to check the websites returned in your search are those pertaining to governmental bodies.

Here are some examples:

UK:

https://www.ncsc.gov.uk
https://www.actionfraud.org.uk/
https://www.cifas.org.uk/
https://www.nationalcrimeagency.gov.uk/what-we-do/crime-threats
    /fraud-and-economic-crime
https://www.met.police.uk/advice/advice-and-information/fa/fraud
    /useful-contacts-for-fraud-cyber-crime-advice/

Australia:

https://www.ag.gov.au/Integrity/counter-fraud/fraud-australia/Pages
    /government-responsibility-fraud.aspx
https://www.pmc.gov.au/who-we-are/accountability-and-reporting
    /fraud-control-and-fraud-reporting
https://www.scamwatch.gov.au/

Germany:

https://www.bafin.de/

Ireland:

https://www.bpfi.ie/news/fraud-publications/
https://www.fraudsmart.ie/personal/fraud-scams/

Italy:

https://cert-agid.gov.it/category/news/

New Zealand:

https://www.ncsc.govt.nz/
https://www.gcsb.govt.nz/our-work/ncsc/

The Netherlands:

https://www.fraudehelpdesk.nl/
https://business.gov.nl/regulation/fraud-deception/
https://www.nctv.nl/themas/cybersecurity
https://www.betaalvereniging.nl/en/safety/fraud-prevention-detection-and-response/

European level:

https://www.europol.europa.eu/about-europol/european-cybercrime-centre-ec3
https://ec.europa.eu/anti-fraud/olaf-and-you/report-fraud_en

USA:

https://us-cert.cisa.gov/ncas/tips
https://www.cisa.gov/publication/stop-think-connect-toolkit
https://www.ic3.gov/

References

Barefoot computing. (n.d.). *Be cybersmart*. https://www.barefootcomputing.org/cyber
Cyber Security Intelligence. (2021). *Ransomware attack on Ireland's health service*. https://www.cybersecurityintelligence.com/blog/ransomware-attack-on-irelands-health-service-5647.html
The European Union Agency for Cybersecurity (ENISA). (2020). *ENISA threat landscape 2020 – ransomware*. https://www.enisa.europa.eu/publications/ransomware
Haveibeenpwned. (n.d.a). *Have I been pwned?* https://haveibeenpwned.com/
Haveibeenpwned. (n.d.b). *Pwned passwords*. https://haveibeenpwned.com/Passwords
Hunt, T. (2021, May 28). *Pwned passwords, open source in the .NET foundation and working with the FBI*. https://www.troyhunt.com/pwned-passwords-open-source-in-the-dot-net-foundation-and-working-with-the-fbi/
Kolb, D. A. (1984). *Experiential learning: Experience as the source of learning and development*. Prentice Hall.
Muhammad, Z. (2021, December 17). *2021 saw record breaking number of double extortion ransomware attacks*. Digital Information World. https://www.digitalinformationworld.com/2021/12/2021-saw-record-breaking-number-of.html
National Cyber Security Centre. (2019, November 15). *Securing your devices*. Crown Copyright. https://www.ncsc.gov.uk/guidance/securing-your-devices
Palmer, D. (2021, June 14). *Ransomware: Russia told to tackle cyber criminals operating from within its borders*. ZDNet. https://www.zdnet.com/article/brazilian-superior-electoral-court-hit-by-major-cyberattack/
Ransomware Task Force. (2021). Prepared by the institute for security and technology. *Combatting Ransomware*. https://securityandtechnology.org/wp-content/uploads/2021/04/IST-Ransomware-Task-Force-Report.pdf
Wiederhold, B. K. (2014). The role of psychology in enhancing cybersecurity. *Cyberpsychology, Behavior, and Social Networking, 17*(3), 131–132. https://doi.org/10.1089/cyber.2014.1502

Afterword

Writing the first book to look at cybersecurity topics specifically for coaches, therapists and all other practitioners of confidential data has been an interesting journey. It is a privilege to bring these important topics up and make them visible, but it is also challenging to be the first to do so and pave the way.

My mission throughout stayed firm to bring over information in a way people can absorb it and apply it here and now. Also important to me has been bringing themes over in a way that the learning may go some way to protecting each reader's private cyber life.

In the year up to this being published, cybercrime has gained more prominence in the media due to the growing number of significant attacks. Being able to use the cyberspace has become fundamental to our lives today, but each time we gain a way to be safer online, there is someone already working on a way around it.

As with many things in life, looking away isn't the solution. Instead, we need to take a positive, solutions-focused and layered approach and be part of our own cybersecurity solutions. As I have imparted through this book, to be cybersecure we do need technology, but it is not the only factor. As a wise friend recently noted to me, it is also about culture, psychology and discipline. Those are all factors that come down to you.

I therefore congratulate you that you are now on your way to becoming a more cybersecure practitioner. Be proud of the awareness you have gained from these pages, do share with your clients (per noted in Chapter 8) how you keep them as safe as possible and – most of all – keep learning!

I welcome hearing about your cyber journey, or your suggestions on what you would like to learn next, in either a new edition or a new volume. Do get in touch! Contact information can be found on: https://www.cybersecurepractitioners.com.

Alexandra J.S. Fouracres

Index

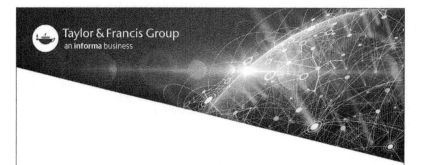